Infectious Diseases

Editor

RANDOLPH F. R. RASCH

NURSING CLINICS
OF NORTH AMERICA

www.nursing.theclinics.com

Consulting Editor
STEPHEN D. KRAU

June 2019 • Volume 54 • Number 2

ELSEVIER

1600 John F. Kennedy Boulevard • Suite 1800 • Philadelphia, Pennsylvania, 19103-2899

http://www.theclinics.com

NURSING CLINICS OF NORTH AMERICA Volume 54, Number 2
June 2019 ISSN 0029-6465, ISBN-13: 978-0-323-67874-2

Editor: Kerry Holland
Developmental Editor: Casey Potter

Nursing Clinics of North America (ISSN 0029-6465) is published quarterly by Elsevier Inc., 360 Park Avenue South, New York, NY 10010-1710. Months of issue are March, June, September, and December. Periodicals postage paid at New York, NY and additional mailing offices. Subscription price per year is, $163.00 (US individuals), $491.00 (US institutions), $275.00 (international individuals), $598.00 (international institutions), $231.00 (Canadian individuals), $598.00 (Canadian institutions), $100.00 (US students), and $135.00 (international students). To receive student/resident rate, orders must be accompanied by name of affiliated institution, date of term, and the signature of program/residency coordinator on institution letterhead. Orders will be billed at individual rate until proof of status is received. Foreign air speed delivery is included in all *Clinics* subscription prices. All prices are subject to change without notice. **POSTMASTER:** Send address changes to *Nursing Clinics*, Elsevier Health Sciences Division, Subscription Customer Service, 3251 Riverport Lane, Maryland Heights, MO 63043. **Customer Service: Telephone: 1-800-654-2452** (U.S. and Canada); **1-314-447-8871 (outside U.S. and Canada). Fax: 1-314-447-8029. E-mail: journalscustomerservice-usa@elsevier.com** (for print support) and **journalsonlinesupport-usa@elsevier.com** (for online support).

Nursing Clinics of North America is covered in *EMBASE/Excerpta Medica, MEDLINE/PubMed (Index Medicus), Social Sciences Citation Index, Current Contents, ASCA, Cumulative Index to Nursing, RNdex Top 100,* and Allied Health Literature and International Nursing Index (INI).

Contributors

CONSULTING EDITOR

STEPHEN D. KRAU, PhD, RN, CNE
Associate Professor (Ret), Vanderbilt University School of Nursing, Nashville, Tennessee

EDITOR

RANDOLPH F. R. RASCH, PhD, RN, FNP, FAANP, FNAP
Dean and Professor, College of Nursing, Michigan State University, East Lansing, Michigan

AUTHORS

TAYLOR A. ARGO, MD
Resident, Department of Pediatrics, University of Minnesota, Minneapolis, Minnesota

ELIZABETH L. BEAM, PhD, RN
Assistant Professor, College of Nursing, University of Nebraska Medical Center, 985330 Nebraska Medical Center, Omaha, Nebraska

KATHLEEN C. BOULTER, MPH, RN
Nurse Manager, Nebraska Biocontainment Unit, Nebraska Medicine, 982470 Nebraska Medical Center, Omaha, Nebraska

AMBER CARRIVEAU, DNP, FNP-BC
Assistant Professor, Family Nurse Practitioner Program Director, Michigan State University College of Nursing, East Lansing, Michigan

THEODORE J. CIESLAK, MD
Associate Professor, Department of Epidemiology, College of Public Health, University of Nebraska Medical Center, 984395 Nebraska Medical Center, Omaha, Nebraska

KAREN DeCOCKER, DNP, APRN, CNM
Assistant Professor, Department of Women, Children, and Family Nursing, College of Nursing, Rush University, Chicago, Illinois

DENISE K. FERRELL, DNP, RN
Associate Dean for Community Engagement and Public Service, Director for Diversity and Inclusion, Assistant Professor, Michigan State University, East Lansing, Michigan

CYNTHIA GERSTENLAUER, ANP-BC, GCNS-BC, CDE, CCD
Nurse Practitioner, Troy Internal Medicine, Troy, Michigan

JANNA R. GEWIRTZ O'BRIEN, MD, FAAP
Adolescent Medicine Fellow, Division of General Pediatrics and Adolescent Health, Department of Pediatrics, University of Minnesota, Minneapolis, Minnesota

JOCELYN J. HERSTEIN, PhD, MPH
Program Coordinator, Global Center for Health Security, University of Nebraska Medical Center, 984388 Nebraska Medical Center, Omaha, Nebraska

ANGELA L. HEWLETT, MD
Associate Professor, Division of Infectious Diseases, Medical Director, Nebraska Biocontainment Unit, Nebraska Medicine, University of Nebraska Medical Center, 985400 Nebraska Medical Center, Omaha, Nebraska

LINDA J. KEILMAN, DNP, GNP-BC, FAANP
Associate Professor, Director, AGPCNP Program, Gerontological Nurse Practitioner, Michigan State University, College of Nursing, Distinguished Educator of Gerontological Nursing (National Hartford Center), East Lansing, Michigan

ANA M. KELLY, PhD, RN
Assistant Professor, School of Nursing, Columbia University, New York, New York

CHRISTOPHER J. KRATOCHVIL, MD
Associate Vice Chancellor for Clinical Research, University of Nebraska Medical Center, Vice President for Research, Nebraska Medicine, 987878 Nebraska Medical Center, Omaha, Nebraska

LUANN LARSON, BSN, RN
Director of Clinical Research Operations, University of Nebraska Medical Center, 986814 Nebraska Medical Center, Omaha, Nebraska

GAYLE B. LOURENS, DNP, MS, CRNA
Director, Nurse Anesthesia Program, Assistant Professor, Michigan State University, East Lansing, Michigan

JOHN J. LOWE, PhD
Assistant Vice Chancellor for Interprofessional Health Security, Associate Professor of Environmental Health, College of Public Health, University of Nebraska Medical Center, 984388 Nebraska Medical Center, Omaha, Nebraska

DONNA BEHLER McARTHUR, PhD, FNP-BC, FAANP, FNAP
Adjunct Clinical Professor, University of Arizona College of Nursing, Department of Neurology, College of Medicine, Tucson, Arizona; Adjunct Professor, Vanderbilt University School of Nursing, Nashville, Tennessee

MICHELLE PARDEE, DNP, FNP-BC
Clinical Assistant Professor, The University of Michigan School of Nursing, Ann Arbor, Michigan

HANNA POOLE, BSN, RN
Graduate Student, Michigan State University College of Nursing, East Lansing, Michigan

MELISSA A. SAFTNER, PhD, CNM, FACNM
Clinical Associate Professor, School of Nursing, University of Minnesota, Minneapolis, Minnesota

MICHELLE M. SCHWEDHELM, MSN, RN
Executive Director, Emergency Management and Biopreparedness, Nebraska Medicine, 987422 Nebraska Medical Center, Omaha, Nebraska

RENEE E. SIEVING, PhD, RN, FAAN, FSAHM
Professor, School of Nursing and Department of Pediatrics, University of Minnesota, Minneapolis, Minnesota

ANNE THOMAS, PhD, ANP-BC, GNP, FAANP
Associate Dean for Academic Affairs, Michigan State University College of Nursing, East Lansing, Michigan

ANGELA M. VASA, BSN, RN
Nurse Manager, Nebraska Biocontainment Unit, Nebraska Medicine, 982470 Nebraska Medical Center, Omaha, Nebraska

Contents

> The 2014 to 2016 Ebola outbreak response resulted in many lessons learned about biocontainment patient care, leading to enhanced domestic capabilities for highly infectious and hazardous communicable diseases. However, additional opportunities for improvement remain. The article identifies and describes key considerations and challenges for laboratory analysis, clinical management, transportation, and personnel management during the care of patients infected with Ebola or other special pathogens. Dedication to maintaining preparedness enables biocontainment patient care teams to perform at the highest levels of safety and confidence.

> Lymphatic filariasis (LF) is a parasitic infection that is spread by mosquitos infected with worm larvae. Several factors will affect the global prevalence of LF in the future. A growing body of evidence suggests that climate change will influence the spread of parasitic diseases and their vectors. Lymphatic filariasis is the leading cause of permanent disfigurement and the second most common cause of long-term disability in the world.

> Drug-resistant tuberculosis (TB) is one of the greatest challenges facing the elimination of TB. In the United States, persons born outside the United States account for 70% of new TB cases. Nucleic acid amplification testing has greatly reduced the amount of time needed for diagnosis of TB, down to 1 to 2 days, compared with waiting 21 days for culture results. The shorter treatment regimen for latent TB infection with weekly isoniazid and rifabutin for 12 weeks provides treatment as effective as the traditional daily isoniazid for 6 months, but with better adherence from patients.

blood and body fluids. Acute hepatitis B and C infections may or may not produce mild symptoms and spontaneously resolve. Some individuals will progress to chronic hepatitis B and C, which can lead to liver fibrosis, cirrhosis, hepatocellular carcinoma, and possibly death. Choosing medications available to treat chronic hepatitis B and C is based on individual serology results, including genotype and level of liver damage. Treatment has been successful in inducing remission and complete recovery in many individuals.

Zika Virus and Pregnancy Concerns 285

Karen DeCocker

Understanding Zika virus (ZIKV) transmission and the risk of birth defects associated with infection during the childbearing years is imperative. Current knowledge helps guide communication, prevention, and planning efforts between health care providers and female patients of childbearing age. Providers must follow updated data and implement ongoing rapid, sensitive, and specific screening and diagnostic testing for ZIKV. Surveillance of infants with known, in utero ZIKV exposure or infection must be maintained to gain a broader understanding of potential defects or injuries that are not immediately obvious at birth and in early infancy.

Emerging Infectious Diseases 297

Donna Behler McArthur

Emerging infectious diseases (EID) and reemerging infectious diseases are increasing globally. Zoonotic diseases are transmitted from animals to humans through direct contact or through food, water, and the environment. Vector-borne diseases are major sources of mortality and morbidity globally. Three mosquito-borne viruses are yellow fever, chikungunya virus, and dengue virus. Recent EIDs include Candida auris, Elizabethkingia anopheles, The Lone Star tick, and avian influenza H7N2. In addition, mcr-1 may contribute to the dissemination of drug resistance to gram-negative bacteria. Nurses play a major role in the identification and prevention of EID within health care settings.

Infectious Diseases

NURSING CLINICS OF NORTH AMERICA

SERIES OF RELATED INTEREST

Critical Care Nursing
Available at: https://www.ccnursing.theclinics.com/

THE CLINICS ARE AVAILABLE ONLINE!
Access your subscription at:
www.theclinics.com

Foreword

Examining Infectious Diseases Through a Social Epidemiologic Perspective

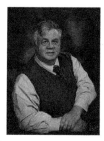

Stephen D. Krau, PhD, RN, CNE
Consulting Editor

When considering infectious diseases, there are many statistics and many pieces of data to consider in relation to trends, incidence, outbreaks, prevention, and the advent of new disease pathogens, to name a few. One recent study by el Bcheraoui and Mokdad identifies that between 1980 and 2014, there were 4,081,546 deaths due to infectious diseases recorded in the United States.[1] It was determined that, in 2014, 113,650 deaths, or a rate of 34.10 deaths per 100,000 persons, were the result of infectious diseases in the United States compared with a total of 72,220 deaths, or a rate of 41.95 deaths per 100,000 persons, in 1980.[1] This identifies an overall decrease of 18.73%. Mortalities from infectious diseases were significantly higher among men than women in all years. Access to data and accuracy of data for countries other than the United States vary, although clear global outbreaks of infectious diseases are well documented and of great concern.

The importance of social factors in health care research and understanding the impact of social factors is essential for the understanding of all disease processes, including infectious diseases. Social factors impact the availability of health care resources, the quality of health care, and overall health and well-being.[2] Essentially, social epidemiology considers the social distribution and social determinants and characteristics that impact the pattern of disease and its distribution. These traits help in the understanding of the mechanisms that occur to enhance and promote disease processes. Some important concepts of social epidemiology include social inequalities, social relationships, social capital, and stress related to work.[3] Although this seems almost common sense to any health care worker, it is has not been a major research focus, particularly in the area of infectious diseases.

https://doi.org/10.1016/j.cnur.2019.03.002
0029-6465/19/© 2019 Published by Elsevier Inc.
nursing.theclinics.com

One need only look at the outbreak of infectious diseases throughout history to examine how these factors have impacted the progression of disease processes from the historical "black plaque," to the advent of AIDS, and the spread of many other diseases, such as tuberculosis, Ebola, and the Zika virus. The focus of much research is on the pathogen itself, the lifecycle of the pathogen, incubation period, means to stop the growth and proliferation of the pathogen, and the identifications of vectors.

SOCIAL INEQUALITY

When considering social epidemiology, one consideration is the factor of "social inequality." With regard to social epidemiology related to infectious diseases, inequalities in health are distinguished from biological differences. Social inequality has been shown to impact health care quality, access, and utilization of health care resources. The impact of disparity of resources and access is the focus of many studies and debate beyond the scope here. However, it is reasonable to draw a correlate between these variables and health care, including incidence and trends of infectious diseases among variant socioeconomic groupings.

SOCIAL RELATIONSHIPS

Social relationships are another factor to be considered in the realm of social epidemiology.

There is evidence suggesting that social relationships impact health care behaviors, such as medical adherence, behaviors that contribute to an individual to seek assistance, and in what manner health care resources are utilized. It has been demonstrated that social support can affect outcomes of medical treatment, such outcomes as recovery, survival, and overall quality of life.[2]

SOCIAL CAPITAL

The concept of "social capital" overlaps with many other phenomena. There is not a clear consensus of the definition of "social capital." Broadly, social capital can be defined as those levels of social structure that include levels of interpersonal trust, norms of reciprocity, civic engagement, and mutual aid. All of these essentially act as resources for individuals and facilitate collective action.[4] The impact between social capital and health care systems as well as patient outcomes is not hard to surmise.

The conceptual framework of social epidemiology provides a theoretical framework to examine and consider all disease processes, including infectious diseases. The factors related to social epidemiology provide a dimension that extends the typical organism, vector-host relationship and introduces new aspects of infectious disease incidence and progression.

Stephen D. Krau, PhD, RN, CNE
Vanderbilt University School of Nursing
6809 Highland Park Drive
Nashville, TN 37206, USA

E-mail address:
steve.krau@vanderbilt.edu

REFERENCES

1. El Bcheraoui C, Mokdad AH, Dwyer-Lindgren L, et al. Trends and patterns of differences in infectious disease mortality among US counties, 1980-2014. JAMA 2018;319(12):1248–60.
2. von dem Knesebeck O. Concepts of social epidemiology in health care research. BMC Health Serv Res 2015;15:357.
3. Berkman LF, Glymour MMKI, editors. Social epidemiology. 2nd edition. Oxford (United Kingdom): Oxford University Press; 2014.
4. Kawachi I, Berkman LF. Social cohesion, social capital and health. In: Berkman LF, Kawachi I, editors. Social epidemiology. Oxford (United Kingdom): Oxford University Press; 2000. p. 174–90.

Preface

Ancient History and New Frontiers: Infectious Diseases

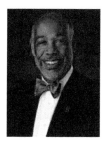

Randolph F.R. Rasch, PhD, RN, FNP, FAANP, FNAP
Editor

As defined by the World Health Organization, "infectious diseases are caused by pathogenic microorganisms, such as bacteria, viruses, parasites or fungi; the diseases can be spread, directly or indirectly, from one person to another."[1] Zoonotic diseases are those that may be spread to humans by animals.[1] The ongoing history, saga, of infectious diseases is a long one. While the concept of infectious disease may be as old as humankind, the idea of what is infectious has changed, considerably, beginning with what was visually unacceptable and moving to what was foul-smelling, until the discovery of microorganisms, the development of germ theory, and the connection between microorganisms and the development of diseases. Infectious diseases are one of the oldest diseases known to humankind.[2] Kelly[3] notes that acid-fast bacilli have been found in pulmonary lesions in human mummies. However, it is unlikely that the Egyptians connected the disease tuberculosis and infection. We do have some indication of the understanding of infectious diseases in ancient times. In a paper discussing the concept of "*tum'ah*" (pollution) in the Hebrew Bible, Feder[4] specifically notes the relationship between pollution and infection, and the association of pollution with genital discharges, corpse pollution, and skin diseases. This pathognomonic association with infectious disease should not surprise us: the idea that a visible change in physical appearance or of contact with something considered unclean, whether or not there was contagious "uncleanness," would lead to disease. Another, historic, way of thinking about infectious disease has been called the Sanitary Era of Epidemiology and is associated with the "ancient miasma theory" of the causation of disease.[5,6] The notion of "miasma" was a key concept in Florence Nightingale's notions about nursing.[7]

The articles appearing in this special infectious disease issue of *Nursing Clinics of North America* reflect our current understandings and provide an update on a range of infectious diseases: their diagnoses, treatment, and the nursing management for

Nurs Clin N Am 54 (2019) xv–xvi
https://doi.org/10.1016/j.cnur.2019.03.001
0029-6465/19/© 2019 Published by Elsevier Inc.

nursing.theclinics.com

infected individuals and individuals closely connected with them. The authors have a range of experience with infectious diseases. Throughout this issue, you will find updated or new concepts around infectious diseases, including lessons learned. These concepts include emerging *new* infectious diseases and emerging *changes* in known infectious diseases; demographics of at-risk individuals and patients, including gender fluidity, and the impact on assessment and treatment; antigenic shifts and antigenic drifts; and genome sequencing for prevention and management. Implications for practice is a theme threaded throughout these articles. With the last article in this issue, surrounding issues of emerging infectious diseases, we come full circle with ancient times. With the melting of glaciers, the possibility of Ice Age bacteria coming to life has given rise to the concern of new infectious diseases from Ice Age microorganisms.[8]

Randolph F.R. Rasch, PhD, RN, FNP, FAANP, FNAP
College of Nursing
Michigan State University
1355 Bogue Street, A216LS
East Lansing, MI 48824, USA

E-mail address:
raschr@msu.edu

REFERENCES

1. World Health Organization. Health topics: infectious diseases. Available at: https://www.who.int/topics/infectious_diseases/en/. Accessed February 16, 2019.
2. Contagion/germ theory/specificity. In: Bynum WF, Porter R, editors. Companion encyclopedia of the history of medicine. Oxford (United Kingdom): Routledge; 2013. p. 309.
3. Kelly AM. Tuberculosis. Nurs Clin N Am 2019;54(2):193–205.
4. Feder Y. Contagion and cognition: bodily experience and the conceptualization of pollution (tum'ah) in the Hebrew Bible. J Near E Stud 2013;72(2):151–67.
5. MacDonald MA. From miasma to fractals: the epidemiology revolution and public health nursing. Public Health Nurs 2004;21(4):380–91.
6. Halliday S. Death and miasma in Victorian London: an obstinate belief. BMJ 2001; 323(7327):1469–72.
7. Nightingale F. 1875: In this manuscript addition Nightingale describes the relationship between air from sewers and disease, and suggests the remedy. In: Skretkowicz V, editor. Notes on nursing and notes on nursing for the laboring classes. Commemorative edition with historical commentary; 2010. p. 420–6.
8. Young K. Ice age bacteria brought back to life. Available at: https://www.newscientist.com/article/dn7064-ice-age-bacteria-brought-back-to-life/downloaded. Accessed February 16, 2019.

Ebola Virus Disease
Clinical Challenges, Recognition, and Management

Elizabeth L. Beam, PhD, RN[a,*], Michelle M. Schwedhelm, MSN, RN[b],
Kathleen C. Boulter, MPH, RN[c], Angela M. Vasa, BSN, RN[c],
LuAnn Larson, BSN, RN[d], Theodore J. Cieslak, MD[e],
John J. Lowe, PhD[f], Jocelyn J. Herstein, PhD, MPH[g],
Christopher J. Kratochvil, MD[h], Angela L. Hewlett, MD[i]

KEYWORDS

- Ebola virus • Biocontainment • Biosecurity • Emerging diseases
- Clinical management

KEY POINTS

- Heightened infection control considerations led to lessons learned for US biocontainment care units that provided care to patients with the Ebola virus disease in 2014 to 2015.
- Protocols for caring for patients with the Ebola virus or other special pathogens should ensure the safety of staff and be well-practiced through trainings and exercises.
- The 2014 to 2016 Ebola outbreak response led to changes in approach and enhanced preparedness for future threats; however, additional opportunities for improvement remain.

Disclosure Statement: The authors report no conflicts of interest and have nothing to disclose.
[a] College of Nursing, University of Nebraska Medical Center, 985330 Nebraska Medical Center, Omaha, NE 68198, USA; [b] Emergency Management and Biopreparedness, Nebraska Medicine, 987422 Nebraska Medical Center, Omaha, NE 68198, USA; [c] Nebraska Biocontainment Unit, Nebraska Medicine, 982470 Nebraska Medical Center, Omaha, NE 68198, USA; [d] University of Nebraska Medical Center, 986814 Nebraska Medical Center, Omaha, NE 68198, USA; [e] Department of Epidemiology, College of Public Health, University of Nebraska Medical Center, 984395 Nebraska Medical Center, Omaha, NE 68198, USA; [f] College of Public Health, University of Nebraska Medical Center, 984388 Nebraska Medical Center, Omaha, NE 68198, USA; [g] Global Center for Health Security, University of Nebraska Medical Center, 984388 Nebraska Medical Center, Omaha, NE 68198, USA; [h] University of Nebraska Medical Center, Nebraska Medicine, 987878 Nebraska Medical Center, Omaha, NE 68198, USA; [i] Division of Infectious Diseases, Nebraska Biocontainment Unit, Nebraska Medicine, University of Nebraska Medical Center, 985400 Nebraska Medical Center, Omaha, NE 68198, USA
* Corresponding author.
E-mail address: ebeam@unmc.edu

Nurs Clin N Am 54 (2019) 169–180
https://doi.org/10.1016/j.cnur.2019.02.001
0029-6465/19/© 2019 Elsevier Inc. All rights reserved.

The epidemic of Ebola virus disease (EVD) in West Africa that began in 2013 was the world's 25th known outbreak of the disease, dwarfing, in numbers of cases, the previous 24 combined. Transmitted from person to person, more than 28,000 people were ultimately infected, and more than 11,000 were killed, with the bulk of the cases in Guinea, Liberia, and Sierra Leone.[1] As local health care systems struggled to respond to the large number of infected patients, health care providers from the United States and other countries responded to the outbreak in Africa through multiple aid organizations. These heroic individuals were faced with providing care to very ill patients with limited clinical resources. The hysteria over EVD in the media and among the state and local agencies responsible for making decisions regarding the monitoring and quarantine of returning health care workers were reminiscent of challenges encountered in the early days of the acquired immunodeficiency syndrome (AIDS) crisis of the 1980s.[2] The media was concurrently attempting to cover the unprecedented outbreak while sharing public policy on the situation throughout the events.[3] In the fall of 2014, a patient who had recently traveled from West Africa was treated at a hospital in the United States. The patient was eventually confirmed to have EVD, ultimately resulting in 2 nurses who had direct contact with the patient also acquiring the illness.[4] EVD is a viral illness with some overlapping symptoms of other common and travel-related illnesses, so educating the public became critical to prevent panic and public concern regarding transmission of the virus (**Fig. 1**).

The Ebola virus is an enveloped RNA virus classified in the Filoviridae family.[5] The typical transmission pattern of the Ebola virus through direct contact with blood, secretions, or tissues of infected humans or nonhuman primates was described in a consensus paper in 2002.[6] At that time, outbreaks of EVD had typically been limited to remote areas of Africa and were controlled without the use of airborne precautions. Despite this, the consensus statement specifically suggested the use of N95 respirators or powered air purifying respirators for respiratory protection to protect health care workers in light of several situations in which transmission could not be fully explained.[6] At the time, the knowledge of EVD and the other viral hemorrhagic fevers was largely limited to primate studies and learnings from outbreak responses.

Recognizing emerging infectious disease threats, key leaders in the United States developed consensus around the establishment of biocontainment units in 2006, detailing aspects such as provision of clinical care, infection control standards, facility design, and ethical issues for high level isolation.[7] Early learnings from the Nebraska Biocontainment Unit were also outlined in the literature and included design priorities, unit management, and challenges in transporting patients.[8] Moreover, the classification of hemorrhagic fever viruses as category A bioweapon agents[6] creates challenges for laboratory recognition and clinical management, specifically specimen shipment and waste handling.[9] Unique regulations and heightened infection control considerations led to many lessons learned for US biocontainment care units that provided patient care to patients with EVD.

The recent West African outbreak was caused by *Zaire ebolavirus*; however, other members of the genus *Ebolavirus*, namely Bundibugyo virus and Sudan virus, would be expected to share transmission modes, produce similar disease, and require similar infection control precautions. The same can be said for the viruses of the genus *Marburgvirus* (along with ebolaviruses, members of the family Filoviridae): Marburg and Ravn. In addition, other viral hemorrhagic fever viruses, such as Lassa, Junin, Machupo, Sabia, Guanarito, and Crimean-Congo, would be expected to produce disease that, although potentially variable in presentation, would also require meticulous attention to personal protection and infection control guidance.

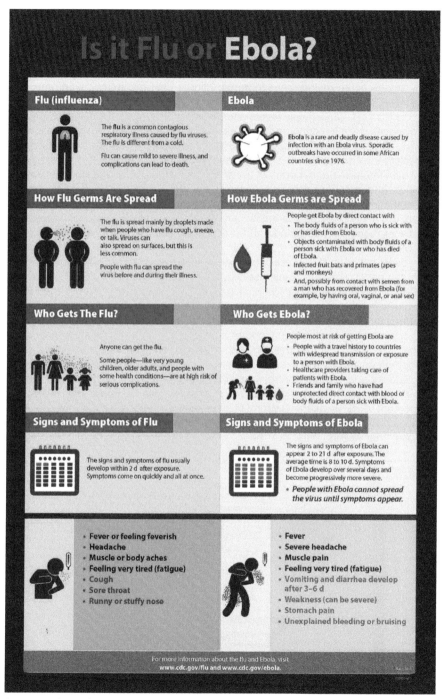

Fig. 1. Is it Flu or Ebola? (*From* CDC. Available at: https://www.cdc.gov/vhf/ebola/pdf/is-it-flu-or-ebola.pdf. Accessed October 8, 2018.)

In addition to the viral hemorrhagic fevers, several other human diseases are known to be highly infectious, highly contagious, and highly hazardous. As such, patients harboring these diseases are considered to be candidates for care in biocontainment units. Included among these are a group of severe acute respiratory diseases thought capable of transmission via droplet nuclei (and thus requiring airborne precautions), namely severe acute respiratory syndrome, Middle East respiratory syndrome, and certain novel, avian, and prepandemic strains of influenza.

Beyond the viral hemorrhagic fevers and severe acute respiratory diseases, several other diseases pose infection control challenges and potentially warrant biocontainment care. Smallpox, monkeypox, Nipah, Hendra, pneumonic plague, and extensively drug-resistant tuberculosis are among these. Although these diseases differ in their clinical manifestations and modes of transmission, and although the infection control modalities and personal protective equipment (PPE) ensembles used to protect against them may also differ, they share a high degree of hazard and communicability. As such, it is imperative that the health care worker caring for patients with these diseases be exceedingly well-trained and practiced in the use of these modalities and ensembles.

Moreover, although the concerning pathogens over time may change or be unknown, the basic modes of transmission will remain the same. The Centers for Disease Control and Prevention's National Institute for Occupational Safety and Health developed a hierarchy of controls designed to prevent injury and illness in the workplace (**Fig. 2**). The hierarchy can be used to guide the development of protocols aimed at protecting health care workers from occupational hazards and exposure. It suggests a ranking of effectiveness with elimination and substitution described as the most effective because they direct removal or replacement of the hazard. This is followed by engineering controls, to isolate people from the hazard, and administration controls, which change the way people work through training or protocol development. PPE is at the bottom of the hierarchy and described as the least effective control. This is not because PPE is ineffective but as a control measure it means the hazard has not been eliminated or replaced, and protection

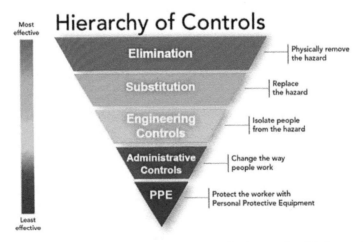

Fig. 2. Hierarchy of controls. (*From* National Institute for Occupational Safety and Health. Available at: https://www.cdc.gov/niosh/topics/hierarchy/default.html. Accessed on October 8, 2018.)

is required.[10] PPE guidelines have been in place in the realm of health care–associated infection and isolation care with little modification for over a decade.[11] Despite this guidance, the lack of standards for design and performance of gowns in particular came to light after the experience of treating patients with EVD in 2014.[12] The Nebraska Biocontainment Unit has described the protocols used for protection of health care workers for EVD care in the literature.[13] The initial standards and procedures set by the hospitals that cared for patients with Ebola in the United States eventually became a guidance resource for managing patients with EVD worldwide.[14]

RECOGNITION

When a disease outbreak occurs, public health and health care systems need to work together to monitor for the emergence of cases and remain vigilant. Because EVD cases were occurring in West Africa in 2014, travel screening was initiated at designated international airports with follow-up from the local public health department for active monitoring of fever or other symptoms.[15] Travel screening was also implemented at health care facilities across the country because an ill patient might present for medical care through the emergency department, ambulatory clinic, or other point of entry to a health care facility.[16] Quick front desk assessment was encouraged to include travel history, travel location, timeframe, and symptoms. This action allowed prompt identification and isolation when appropriate until further discernment could be made to drive laboratory testing decisions. Integrating this strategy into the electronic health record hard wired the process and alerted other caregivers if travel and symptom screening triggered an alert. Creation of consistent work flow and process tools for use by caregivers at all entry areas allowed for consistency in whom to contact, the type of isolation needed, the location of PPE, and various other duties or actions to take (**Fig. 3**).

The Centers for Disease Control and Prevention and the Health and Human Services Assistant Secretary for Preparedness and Response (ASPR) developed a tiered approach to preparedness for EVD (**Fig. 4**), which includes regional Ebola and other special pathogen treatment centers, state designated EVD treatment centers, state designated EVD assessment hospitals, and frontline health care facilities.[15] Frontline

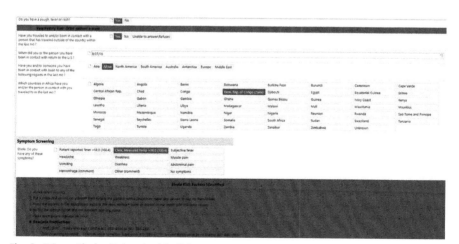

Fig. 3. Triage Ebola: Nebraska Medicine.

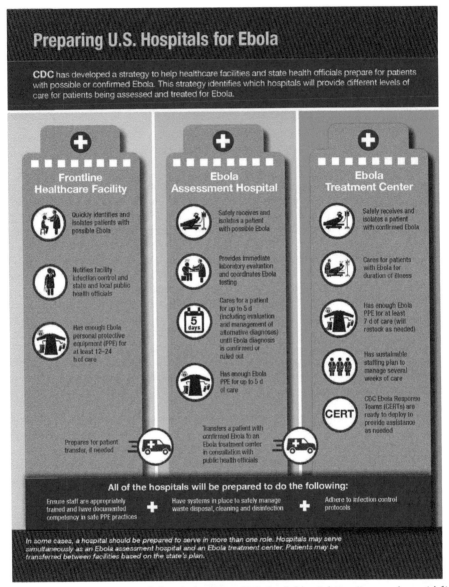

Fig. 4. Preparing U.S. Hospitals for Ebola. (*From* CDC. Available at: https://www.cdc.gov/vhf/ebola/pdf/preparing-hospitals-ebola-P.pdf. Accessed October 8, 2018.)

health care facilities include any facility not otherwise designated as a higher tier and also include emergency departments and other urgent care settings that are expected to safely and effectively identify potential cases, isolate those individuals in a timely manner, and inform the appropriate public health officials (**Fig. 5**). Ebola assessment hospitals are expected to care for patients under investigation until a diagnosis can be confirmed or ruled out. If confirmed, a patient would be transferred to a regional or state designated Ebola treatment center, which is expected to provide care for the duration of the patient's illness.[15]

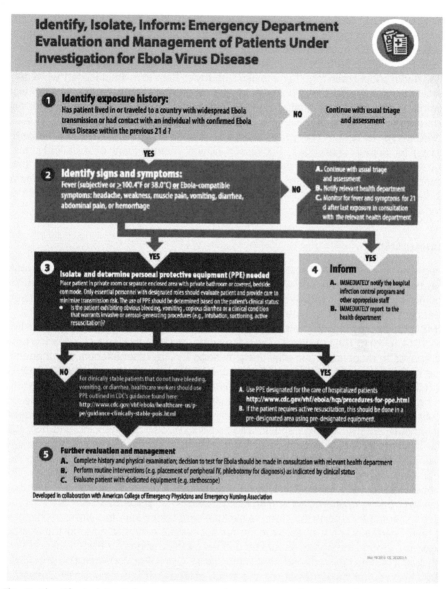

Fig. 5. Identify, isolate, inform: emergency department evaluation and management of patients under investigation for Ebola virus disease. (*From* CDC. Available at: https://www.cdc.gov/vhf/ebola/pdf/ed-algorithm-management-patients-possible-ebola.pdf. Accessed on October 8, 2018.)

Laboratory resources are a critical element of both a recognition and management plan for patients with EVD. Public health laboratories in the Laboratory Response Network are authorized to perform the molecular screening test for EVD.[17] Risk assessment is a critical element of developing a laboratory plan for EVD testing, and the Association of Public Health Laboratories has developed a template for this process.[18] Laboratories use a combination of point-of-care testing and compact analyzers that fit into a biosafety cabinet, as well as large automated closed-tube an-alyzers in core testing facilities.[19] When preparing a laboratory to support the care of patients with EVD, a specialized and trained team should be assembled, and a safe space identified to perform the testing. A test menu should be established. The labo-ratory team should train together and use a buddy system to maintain safety while per-forming testing. The laboratorians should practice routine skills and run laboratory test controls in the space designated for EVD testing to develop muscle memory for the different skills and clinical challenges that they will face when working with specimens in PPE that is not used in everyday practice. Practicing these skills allows for problem-solving for unique challenges. Successful clinical management of a patient under investigation or a confirmed patient with EVD will depend on a collaborative and connected relationship between the physician team, the nursing team, and the clinical laboratorians, with a strong connection to public health laboratories throughout the process.

MANAGEMENT

If a patient is not identified in close proximity to an assessment or treatment center, they may need to be transported from another state in the region, or even from another country outside the United States, to receive care at a regional or state designated treatment center.[15] This type of transport requires emergency medical service (EMS) provided by trained professionals to support transportation of the patient. After the 2014 to 2016 EVD outbreak, federal funding became available to advance pre-paredness to respond to and effectively manage EVD or other infectious pathogens. One of the requests for all states was to create a concept of operations (CONOPs) to include, at a minimum, a plan to coordinate air or ground transport within the state and region. Direction, control, and coordination are described in detail to guide an event response. Anticipated key participating agencies must agree to the process that is outlined. These plans should also specifically discuss financing and how the plan itself is maintained through training and exercises. A critical element in prepared-ness planning includes exercising the plan to allow for refinement and ensuring the operational capability of a written plan. Forming a training and exercise planning com-mittee can provide a venue to increase engagement across all partners and further develop working relationships among key partners. During the activation of a regional network, some transports may require multiple care teams and, therefore, exchanges of team members, as well as refueling for successful extended ground transports. Extended ground transports should be defined by the designated EMS transport ser-vice and the state health department in the state's CONOPs. Consideration should be given to the condition of the patient, the length of time staff can remain in PPE, and the distance the EMS vehicle can travel before needing to refuel. This type of coordinated trip requires advance planning and creative thinking to identify safe locations to perform these tasks. Many regions are exercising their regional plans and working through these challenges. These types of exercises to advance regional planning focus on the communication processes, patient care handoffs and the importance of the connection between EMS and nursing. Clinical updates during the transport and at the point of transition are critical to continuous quality care of the patient.

The decision to transport a patient with EVD is difficult. The risk involved in caring for the patient increases on leaving the relative safety of a controlled clinical care environ-ment in a hospital setting for the fluid, less stable setting of ground or air transportation vehicles. As such, transportation may require clinical management that operates un-der altered standards of care. As a precaution for any potential generation of aerosols that may affect the driver during ground transport, air handling in the transport vehicle is set to prevent the circulation of air, with the ventilation fan put on high in the driver's compartment to establish a positive-pressure environment.[20] Decisions on the amount of barrier protection required for a ground vehicle transport and for the preparation of the patient should be made well in advance. Some teams use 6-mil plastic sheeting to create these barriers in the patient care area,[19] whereas others have identified prefabricated enclosures or have purchased purpose-built ambulances. If barriers are used, materials will add to the waste burden on arrival to the destination. Cooperative patients may tolerate an impervious suit and mask, whereas others may be unresponsive or unable to adequately control bodily fluids and require a more reliable containment device or wrap.[20] Many of these same challenges exist in the aircraft environment, with additional concerns related to the safety regulations for flight. Limitations exist on the type of chemical disinfectants that can be used so as not to compromise airworthiness (eg, not deteriorate aircraft components), and materials for restraint, such as seat belts or airline seats, are difficult to decontaminate. Moreover, certain electronic equipment routinely used in a ground vehicle or hospital environment may be prohibited on an aircraft due to interference of wireless services. Also, medical equipment must be deemed safe-to-fly by the appropriate authority. Guidance is available on many of these issues specific to the air medical transport of patients with EVD.[21] The high-risk nature of such transports demands clear lines of communication between transport teams and referring and receiving facilities, including frequent, accurate updates by transporting EMS teams on clinical status. Communicating the estimated time of arrival and patient information helps to establish receiving teams' expectations to facilitate timely, successful patient transitions. On arrival at the receiving hospital, a team of isolation unit staff, wearing appropriate PPE and trained in decontamination protocols, should meet the ground transport vehicle. Any fluid spills should be immediately decontaminated, followed by a full decontamination of the intrafacility route on patient placement. The full decontamination process is performed for community reassurance, especially in situations in which the transport occurs in public spaces.

After the patient is safely transported to the hospital, providing care to a patient with confirmed EVD requires more resources than a typical hospitalized patient owing to the rigorous safety controls and the specialized team required to successfully care for a patient in a biocontainment unit.[21] Protocols should be developed that direct the management of the unit and ensure the safety of staff, and these should be practiced through trainings and exercises. Protocols are refined based on feedback from the staff, which promotes ownership of the plans. Protocols should also be reviewed by an interprofessional team with expertise in all facets of the process. For example, a provider-down protocol directs the plan to get an ill or incapacitated health care worker out of the patient care room, out of PPE, and provide them with the required medical care. Other protocols might include staff monitoring or symptom surveillance, spill cleanup, and care of the deceased patient.

The disease severity of the patients with EVD cared for in the United States and Europe ranged from moderate to critical, with some patients developing complications that resulted in death.[22] Caring for a patient with EVD requires nursing staff be skilled and proficient in the care of patients for all stages of their illness. Some biocontainment units use nursing staff from many specialties to include critical care, medical-surgical, pediatrics, procedural services, and others to obtain a skill-mix, whereas other teams are made up solely of critical care nurses. Respiratory therapists (RTs) and patient care technicians can provide additional support. Education and training of the team is an ongoing cycle and consists of PPE donning and doffing, operating specialized equipment in the unit, practicing hands-on clinical skills while in PPE, infection control training, and education on infectious diseases and current outbreaks. A training and exercise plan should include quarterly drills with other agencies or departments within the hospital and the community.

Staffing is best explained with a case study. During the activations in 2014 to 2016, when caring for a single EVD patient, the Nebraska Biocontainment Unit operated with 6 staff members on the day shift and 5 staff members on the night shift. Each shift included at least 3 registered nurses. If the patient was in need of respiratory care, an RT was also present. Each staff member was assigned a staffing role at the beginning of each shift with specific tasks and everyone rotated through the roles, remaining within their scope of practice. The 3 registered nurses assigned to patient care worked directly at the patient's bedside in 4-hour shifts. Generally, 1 registered nurse was in the patient care room but this number increased in critically ill patients who required intensive care. Staffing depends on multiple factors, such as the number of patients that can be cared for, patient acuity, and the physical structure of a biocontainment unit.

Procedures in a biocontainment unit must be performed in a controlled and coordinated manner to enhance safety of the patient and health care workers. Central venous catheter insertion is performed to facilitate phlebotomy and provide intravenous access for medications and fluids. Intubation is performed using rapid sequence induction to reduce the creation of aerosols, patient movement, or reflexes such as coughing. The use of a video laryngoscope allows the physician to distance themselves from the patient's airway.[23] Patients with EVD commonly develop copious amounts of diarrhea that can lead to dehydration and this alone or in combination with sepsis sequelae can result in acute kidney injury, so considerations and planning to provide dialysis or continuous renal replacement therapy (CRRT) is essential.[23] In regard to renal replacement, processes for cleaning the equipment, ensuring safety of the lines, and treating the effluent must be developed.[22] Studies investigating the effluent from CRRT found no viral material present, suggesting the virus does not cross the dialyzer membrane[24]; however, precautions are still advised.

Because no treatment of EVD approved by the US Food and Drug Administration is available, various investigational therapeutic agents were used in the management of patients with EVD during the 2014 to 2016 outbreak. Investigational therapeutics were administered to people who experienced a high-risk exposure, as well as patients with confirmed EVD. Unfortunately, the uncontrolled nature of the open-label use in most instances and the limited numbers of individuals treated with experimental therapeutics, as well as the use of multiple concomitant investigational products simultaneously, made generalization of the data challenging.[25,26] In response to this unmet need, the Special Pathogens Research Network (SPRN) was organized after the 2014 to 2016 outbreak to proactively develop a centralized infrastructure to initiate research protocols and collect meaningful data. Sponsored by ASPR, this network of 10 regional treatment centers supported by centralized research resources such as a biorepository, data repository, case report forms, and a central rapid response institutional review board, will help to efficiently and systematically launch research protocols in the next outbreak. This readiness is further ensured by routine regional and national exercises involving the SPRN and the 10 regional centers.

The 2014 to 2016 Ebola outbreak response resulted in many lessons learned, leading to changes in approach and preparedness; however, additional opportunities for improvement remain. Key challenges in laboratory analysis, waste management, clinical management, research, and workforce issues persist.[27] Multidisciplinary teamwork is critical to address the unique problem solving challenges of caring for patients infected with Ebola or other special pathogens, and dedication to maintenance of preparedness allow these teams able to perform at the highest levels of safety and confidence.[28]

REFERENCES

1. WHO Ebola Response Team. After Ebola in West Africa: unpredictable risks, preventable epidemics. N Engl J Med 2016;375:587–96.
2. Gonsalves G, Staley P. Panic, paranoia, and public health: the AIDS epidemic's lessons for Ebola. N Engl J Med 2014;371:2348–9.
3. Sell TK, Boddie C, McGinty EE, et al. News media coverage of US Ebola policies: implications for communication during future infectious disease threats. Prev Med 2016;93:15–120.
4. Liddell AM, Davey RT, Mehta AK, et al. Characteristics and clinical management of a cluster of 3 patients with Ebola virus disease, including the first domestically acquired cases in the United States. Ann Intern Med 2015;163:81–91.
5. Kiley MP, Bowen ET, Eddy GA, et al. Filoviridae: a taxonomic home for Marburg and Ebola viruses? Intervirology 1982;18:24–32.
6. Borio L, Inglesby T, Peters CJ, et al. Hemorrhagic fever viruses as biological weapons: medical and public health management. JAMA 2002;287:2391–405.
7. Smith PW, Anderson AO, Christopher GW, et al. Designing a biocontainment unit to care for patients with serious communicable diseases: a consensus statement. Biosecur Bioterror 2006;4:351–65.
8. Beam EL, Boulter KC, Freihaut F, et al. The Nebraska experience in biocontainment patient care. Public Health Nurs 2010;27:140–7.
9. Hewlett AL, Varkey JB, Smith PW, et al. Ebola virus disease: preparedness and infection control lessons learned from two biocontainment units. Curr Opin Infect Dis 2015;28:343–8.
10. National Institute for Occupational Safety and Health. Hierarchy of controls. 2018. Available at: https://www.cdc.gov/niosh/topics/hierarchy/default.html. Accessed October 15, 2018.
11. Centers for Disease Control and Prevention. Protecting healthcare personnel. 2016. Available at: https://www.cdc.gov/hai/prevent/ppe.html. Accessed October 15, 2018.
12. Kilinc Balci FS. Isolation gowns in health care settings: Laboratory studies, regulations and standards, and potential barriers of gown selection and use. Am J Infect Control 2016;44:104–11.
13. Beam EL, Schwedhelm S, Boulter K, et al. Personal protective equipment processes and rationale for the Nebraska Biocontainment Unit during the 2014 activations for Ebola virus disease. Am J Infect Control 2016;44:340–2.
14. Centers for Disease Control and Prevention. Guidance on personal protective equipment (PPE) to be used by healthcare workers during management of patients with confirmed Ebola or persons under investigation (PUIs) for Ebola who are clinically unstable or have bleeding, vomiting, or diarrhea in U.S. hospitals, including procedures for donning and doffing PPE. 2015. Available at: https://www.cdc.gov/vhf/ebola/healthcare-us/ppe/guidance.html. Accessed October 15, 2018.
15. Koonin LM, Jamieson DJ, Jernigan JA, et al. Systems for rapidly detecting and treating persons with Ebola virus disease – United States. MMWR Morb Mortal Wkly Rep 2015;64:222–5.

16. Schwedhelm S, Swanhorst J, Watson S, et al. ED Ebola triage algorithm: a tool and process for compliance. J Emerg Nurs 2015;41(2):165–9.

17. Wadman MC, Schwedhelm SS, Watson S, et al. Emergency department processes for the evaluation and management of persons under investigation for Ebola virus disease. Ann Emerg Med 2015;66:306–14.

18. Association of Public Health Laboratories. Template for public health laboratory risk assessment for Ebola Virus Disease (EVD) testing. Available at: https://www.aphl.org/programs/preparedness/Documents/APHL-Template.pdf. Accessed July 3, 2018.

19. Herstein JJ, Iwen PC, Jelden KC, et al. U. S. High-level isolation unit clinical laboratory capabilities update. J Clin Microbiol 2018;56 [pii:e01608-17].

20. Isakov A, Miles W, Gibbs S, et al. Transport and management of patients with confirmed or suspected Ebola virus disease. Ann Emerg Med 2015;66:297–305.

21. Centers for Disease Control and Prevention. Guidance on Air Medical Transport (AMT) for patients with Ebola Virus Disease (EVD). Available at: https://www.cdc.gov/vhf/ebola/clinicians/emergency-services/air-medical-transport.html. Accessed August 1, 2018.

22. Uyeki TM, Mehta AK, Davey RT, et al. Clinical management of Ebola virus disease in the United States and Europe. N Engl J Med 2016;374:636–46.

23. Vasa A, Schwedhelm M, Johnson D. Critical care for the patient with Ebola Virus Disease: the Nebraska perspective. J Intensive Crit Care 2015;1:1–5.

24. Connor MJ, Kraft C, Mehta AK, et al. Successful delivery of RRT in Ebola virus disease. J Am Soc Nephrol 2015;26:31–7.

25. Kraft CS, Hewlett AL, Koepsell S, et al. The use of TKM-100802 and convalescent plasma in 2 patients with Ebola Virus Disease in the United States. Clin Infect Dis 2015;61:496–502.

26. Wong KK, Davey RT, Hewlett AL, et al. Use of postexposure prophylaxis after occupational exposure to *Zaire ebolavirus*. Clin Infect Dis 2016;63:376–9.

27. Meyer D, Sell TK, Schoch-Spana M, et al. Lessons from the domestic Ebola response: Improving health care system resilience to high consequence infectious diseases. Am J Infect Control 2018;46:533–7.

28. Schwedhelm S, Beam EL, Morris RD, et al. Reflections on interprofessional team-based clinical care in the ebola epidemic: The Nebraska Medicine experience. Nurs Outlook 2015;63:27–9.

Lymphatic Filariasis

Gayle B. Lourens, DNP, MS, CRNA[a],*, Denise K. Ferrell, DNP, RN[b]

KEYWORDS

- Lymphatic filariasis • Parasite • Mosquito • Larvae

KEY POINTS

- Lymphatic filariasis (LF) is a parasitic infection that is spread by mosquitoes infected with worm larvae.
- LF is the leading cause of permanent disfigurement and the second most common cause of long-term disability in the world.
- The World Health Organization provides guidelines and protocols for drug treatment, symptom management, disease mapping and monitoring and evaluating outcomes.
- Several factors will effect the global prevalence of LF in the future including climate change and population migration.

INTRODUCTION AND EPIDEMIOLOGY

Lymphatic filariasis (LF) is a parasitic infection that is spread by mosquitos infected with worm larvae. Classified as a neglected tropical disease by the World Health Organization (WHO), Centers for Disease Control and Prevention, and the National Institute of Allergy and Infectious Diseases, this incurable condition affects more than 120 million people worldwide.[1–3] An endemic disease in 73 countries, 1.1 billion people are at risk of exposure to and contracting the infectious disease in the tropical and subtropical regions of Asia, Africa, the western Pacific, and parts of South America and the Caribbean.[4]

In 1997, the WHO classified the disease as eradicable or potentially eradicable and passed a resolution to eliminate the parasitic infection by the year 2020. With several new advances in diagnostics, pharmaceutical treatment options, and the formation of the Global Program to Eliminate Lymphatic Filariasis (GPELF), WHO member states were presented with a strategic plan consisting of 2 goals: interrupt the transmission and spread of LF through mass drug administration (MDA) and alleviate suffering for those with LF-related chronic conditions.[5]

LF is the leading cause of permanent disfigurement and the second most common cause of long-term disability in the world. Forty million people are disfigured and

[a] Michigan State University, 1355 Bogue Street, East Lansing, MI 48824, USA; [b] Michigan State University, 1355 Bogue Street, East Lansing, MI 48824, USA
* Corresponding author.
E-mail address: loniews8@msu.edu

Nurs Clin N Am 54 (2019) 181–192
https://doi.org/10.1016/j.cnur.2019.02.007
0029-6465/19/© 2019 Elsevier Inc. All rights reserved.

disabled by the disease, making it an important public health and socioeconomic problem.[6] Although MDA has had a major impact on the spread of the disease in several countries, less progress has been made in alleviating the suffering for those already infected with the condition.[7]

TRANSMISSION

Wuchereria bancrofti (WB), *Brugia malayi*, and *Brugia timori* are three closely related nematode worms responsible for LF. Of these, humans are the exclusive host for WB, which is responsible for 90% of all LF cases worldwide. The transmission cycle begins when an infected female mosquito bites and deposits LF larvae on the skin (**Fig. 1**).[8] The larvae enter the bite wound and travel to the lymphatic vessels. Over the course of 6 to 12 months, they mature into adult male and female worms. During her 7-year life cycle, the female can release up to 10,000 embryonic offspring (microfilaria) per day. The microfilariae (Mf) are carried by the natural lymph flow and are introduced into the blood. When the human host is awake, Mf preferentially remain in the larger blood vessels; however, during sleep, they travel to surface vessels, enabling them to be ingested by night-biting mosquitos. In the mosquito, the Mf undergo several stages of molting and development. The larvae are ready for human transmission in 10 to 12 days.[4,9]

The circadian periodicity of Mf activity, although nocturnal in many parts of the world, seems to coordinate with the carrier mosquito's sleep-wake cycle. For example, in the Pacific Islands, diurnal periodicity is most common. From a practical point of view, knowing the periodicity informs blood collection times and enhances the accuracy of diagnosis.[10]

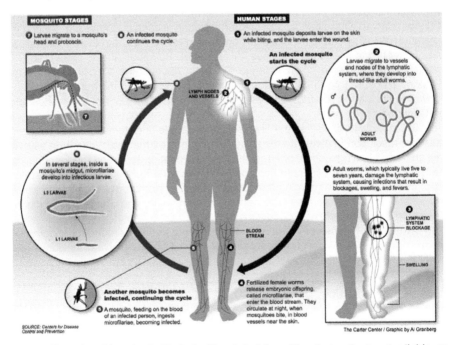

Fig. 1. Life cycle of lymphatic filariasis. (*Reprinted from* The Carter Center. Available at: https://www.cartercenter.org/resources/pdfs/health/lf/lymphatic-filariasis-life-cycle.pdf. Accessed September 1, 2018; with permission.)

Transmission in a community is influenced by several factors: the prevalence or number of infected persons, the density of Mf in the blood of the infected person, the density of carrying mosquitos in the endemic region, characteristics that affect the growth and development of the larvae, and frequency of human contact with the infected mosquitos.[4,11]

Repeated mosquito bites over several months are needed to contract LF.[6] Thus, natives or long-term visitors residing within endemic areas are at the greatest risk.[7] Once thought to be an adult disease, it has become increasingly apparent that transmission primarily occurs in childhood, with clinical manifestations presenting in young or older adults.[12]

PATHOGENESIS

In healthy individuals, lymphatic vessels remove circulating fluid and large molecules, such as proteins, from the extracellular space of nearly every body tissue. The lymph system is essential for maintaining a correct extracellular fluid volume and clearing pathogens that have crossed the skin barrier and entered the extravascular compartments. Antigens, pathogens, and macrophage-engulfed invaders are afferently transported to the lymph nodes to undergo adaptive immunity processes and removal. Once cleaned and filtered, the lymph fluid is returned to the vascular space.[13]

As a component of the adaptive immune system, T lymphocytes are programmed to recognize, respond to, and remember foreign antigens. The presence of cell surface molecules known as CD4 or CD8 distinguishes T lymphocytes. CD4 T lymphocytes, also called helper T (Th) cells, are prolific cytokine producers. Cytokines are hormonal messengers within the immune system and are responsible for cell-mediated immune and allergic responses, thus they are often grouped as either proinflammatory (Th1 response) or antiinflammatory (Th2 response).[14]

In LF, damage to the lymphatic vessels is mediated by a response to the presence of the adult worm and products released by the worm. Compounds secreted or excreted by the live worms act on endothelial cells, causing lymph tissue scarring, gradual loss of lymphatic vessel contractility, destruction of the unidirectional valves, and lymphangiectasis (a pathologic dilatation of lymph vessels). Regardless of treatment, the damage to the lymph system is permanent.[15]

On histology, live Mf and the adult worms rarely elicit an immune response. However, dead or dying Mf and adult worms are highly antigenic. Although the mechanism is not fully understood, LF antigens guarantee species survival by modulating the host's immune system (**Fig. 2**) to favor an antiinflammatory (Th2) response. This response is accomplished by reducing the proinflammatory (Th1) response.[16] As result of dampening the immune system, there is a profoundly diminished response to opportunistic pathogens and vaccines, such as tetanus toxoid, which becomes a significant contributor to poor outcomes associated with chronic lymphedema.[17]

Children born to infected mothers are more susceptible to acquiring filarial infections. In women treated with multiple rounds of antifilarial drugs before pregnancy, the incidence of a child acquiring LF is reduced to less than 1%.[18] It is hypothesized that the placental transfer of antigens modulates the infant's immune system, favoring a TH-2 response.[19] Thus, these results support the need for reproductive education and MDA treatment in adolescent girls in endemic areas before pregnancy.

An individual's response to adult worm and Mf presence varies; some develop clinical symptoms and others do not. The cause of these diverse responses is not fully understood. Susceptibility, parasitic load, and the degree of pathologic changes cluster

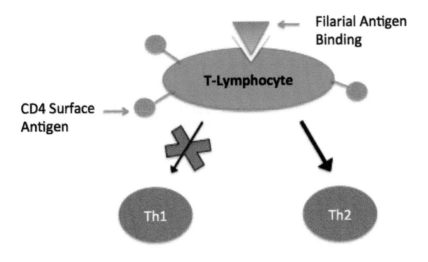

Fig. 2. Antiinflammatory (Th2) pathway following filarial antigen binding. (*Courtesy of Gayle B. Lourens, DNP, MS, CRNA.*)

in families, suggesting genetic polymorphism plays a role in lymph tissue remodeling, severity of lymphatic dysfunction, and degree of immune modulation.[20,21]

To effectively distribute resources and monitor treatment responses, individuals are frequently categorized as:

- Exposed but uninfected
- Infected but clinically asymptomatic
- Acquired acute filarial disease with or without Mf presence (carriers)
- Acquired chronic filarial infection with pathologic conditions[22]

DIAGNOSIS

The WHO provides guidelines and protocols for mapping, monitoring, and evaluating LF programs. The standard method for diagnosing active LF is the identification of Mf presence in a blood smear by a microscopic examination. The presence of Mf on the slide sample depends on the parasitic cycle, sparseness of the organism on the slide, and technician training. Blood collection for the various Mf species requires time-sensitive collection and evaluation. For example, WB Mf are most active between 10 PM and 2 AM[23]

In 1996, the point-of-care immunochromatographic card test (ICT), detecting filarial antigens, was introduced, simplifying diagnosis. In 2000, filarial antigen testing was integrated into the GPELF protocol for mapping endemicity, discontinuation of MDA therapy, and post-MDA surveillance.[24] However, the ICT has a short (3-month) shelf life, requires cold storage, is costly, and is associated with false-positives if read outside of the manufacturer's recommended time frame of 10 minutes.[25] Moreover, recent studies suggest a loss of ICT sensitivity for LF diagnosis in low-prevalence settings. A reduced sensitivity has implications for current processes used to define endemic borders (mapping) and monitor MDA effectiveness.[26]

To address the limitations of ICT, the Bill and Melinda Gates Foundation funded research efforts to develop an improved point-of-care test. The antigen-detecting Alere Filariasis Test Strip (FTS) was added to the GPELF guidelines in 2015.[27] Benefits of FTS include a longer shelf life, better temperature stability, and cost reduction.[28] A growing body of research suggests FTS provides superior sensitivity (accurate detection of lower levels of filarial antigens) to ICT.[29]

Laboratory-based serum tests include enzyme-linked immunosorbent assays (ELISAs), which detect antifilarial IgG4 antibodies. With a reported sensitivity of greater than 95%, and a specificity greater than 94%, positive point-of-care tests are ideally confirmed by ELISA testing. However, the barriers (storage, training, and cost) of ELISAs are often prohibitive.[30] Note that IgG4 antibodies remain present for 1 to 2 years after antifilarial treatment and Mf disappearance, which produces a false-positive test result.[31]

Ultrasonography (US) is the imaging method of choice for detecting the presence of adult worms or worm nests in the pelvic and scrotal lymphatic systems. The worms' twirling movements produce the echogenic, classic filarial dance sign.[32] US is used as a rapid diagnostic tool to rule out LF presence in less common anatomic areas, such as the breast or neck, and aids in the identification of patients requiring immediate surgical intervention. The detectable number of worm nests statistically correlates with the Mf load and circulating antigen levels.[33]

DISEASE PROGRESSION AND SYMPTOMS

Most infected persons are asymptomatic despite circulating Mf or filarial antigen presence. However, most asymptomatic individuals have underlying lymphatic damage.[13] As the diseases progresses (**Fig. 3**), lymphedema develops. Lymph stagnation provides a medium for secondary infective pathogens. Secondary infections are the most important contributor to LF disability and drive acute attacks of dermatolymphangioadenitis (ADLA). Characterized by a sudden onset of fever, severe pain, and swollen limbs or genitalia, ADLA amplifies the presence of lymphedema, which in turn potentiates ADLA, forming a perpetual cycle.[15] Left untreated, elephantiasis develops, which is identified by a grossly enlarge, edematous body part rendering an individual disfigured and permanently disabled. The skin of the affected body part takes on a dry, thick, dark appearance. Wartlike protuberances, containing dilated loops of lymph vessels, form. The edematous, redundant skin folds and skin lesion provide an environment and conduit for secondary infections.[34]

Filarial hydroceles are the most common chronic manifestation in men. Gradual accumulation of fluid in the tunica vaginalis of the scrotal sac is often accompanied by thickening of the spermatic cord and changes in the scrotal skin and subcutaneous tissue. Left untreated, it may lead to other urologic complications, such as lymph scrotum, elephantiasis of the scrotum, inguinal adenitis, and opportunistic infections. Affected individuals often avoid seeking treatment for fear of drawing attention to their condition. The social impact and often silent burden associated with stigmatization directly correlates with the severity of visible disease.[34]

LF is associated with a variety of renal abnormalities, including hematuria, proteinuria, nephrotic syndrome, and glomerulonephritis. Circulating immune complexes containing filarial antigens have been implicated in renal damage. As the lymphatic vessels progressively become inflamed and blocked, lymph vessels become congested. Fistulas within the renal system form, allowing the flow of lymph directly into the urine (chyluria). The milky chyle contains fat, protein, and coagulated fibrin. Clinically, the loss of these essential components leads to fatigue, pain from urethral

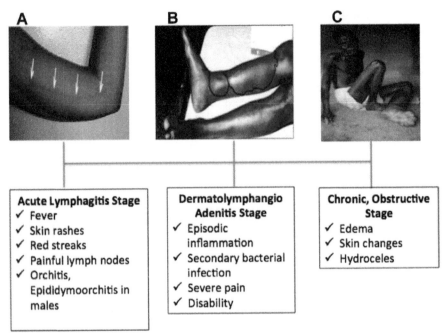

A **B** **C**

Acute Lymphagitis Stage	Dermatolymphangio Adenitis Stage	Chronic, Obstructive Stage
✓ Fever ✓ Skin rashes ✓ Red streaks ✓ Painful lymph nodes ✓ Orchitis, Epididymoorchitis in males	✓ Episodic inflammation ✓ Secondary bacterial infection ✓ Severe pain ✓ Disability	✓ Edema ✓ Skin changes ✓ Hydroceles

Fig. 3. Progression of lymphatic filariasis. (*Reprinted from* [*A, B*] Bennuru S, Babu S, Nutman TB. Etiology and pathophysiology. In: Lee BB, Rockson SG, editors. Lymphedema: a concise compendium of theory and practice. 2nd edition. Cham (Switzerland): Springer International Publishing AG; 2018; with permission; and [*C*] World Health Organization. Available at: http://www.who.int/lymphatic_filariasis/resources/photo_gallery/en/.)

obstruction, and social isolation. The primary treatment of chyluria is treating the LF parasitic infection. The success rate with MDA treatment and a high-protein, reduced-fat diet is approximately 60%. Patients not responding to drug treatment require invasive surgical procedures, such as sclerotherapy (sclerosis of lymphatic renal fistula) and nephrolympholysis (pyelolymphatic disconnection).[35]

Trapped Mf in the pulmonary beds release antigens, causing a localized inflammation. Depicted as significantly high eosinophil serum levels (>3000 µL), tropical pulmonary eosinophilia is a syndrome found mostly in young men between the ages of 15 and 40 years. The associated nightly nonproductive cough and wheezing are likely related to the nocturnal activity of the Mf. This condition is often misdiagnosed as bronchial asthma.[36] The main radiological feature is nodular shadows similar to tuberculosis.[37] Pulmonary function tests show mixed restrictive and obstructive abnormalities. Despite treatment with MDA, 20% of patients may relapse. Although steroids have been shown to be beneficial, exact dosing and treatment protocols are lacking.[36]

DISEASE MANAGEMENT: MASS DRUG ADMINISTRATION

The main treatment of LF is the use of preventive chemotherapy (antiparasitic) drugs administered to the entire at-risk population. These agents reduce the density of the Mf in the blood, thus preventing the transmission to the mosquito. To achieve interruption of parasite transmission in areas with high Mf prevalence, an MDA program must achieve coverage of at least 80% of the target population. Based on the reproductive life span of LF, drug coverage must be given over 5 to 6 consecutive years. MDA strategies (drug combination regimens, dose, and frequency) have been modified as the LF body of scientific evidence has expanded. At present, 1 of 3 drug combinations is administered biannually: albendazole (ALB) plus diethylcarbamazine (DEC), ALB plus ivermectin, or ALB.[38]

Coinfection with other parasites is a factor in MDA management (**Table 1**). DEC has been shown to worsen eye disease in patients coinfected with LF and onchocerciasis (river blindness), caused by a worm that resides in the eye and skin. Likewise, DEC is not recommended for individuals coinfected with LF and loiasis (African eye worm).[39] Quantification of LF Mf is necessary before choosing a drug regimen. Administration of DEC in individuals with significant Mf (>2000 Mf/mL) may cause severe encephalopathy associated with a poor prognosis following DEC administration. Because Mf quantification is often not possible with point-of-care testing, GPELF guidelines recommend ALB biannually. The end points for MDA are Mf levels less than 1% or antigen presence in less than 2% of the target population.[38] LF is a disease that carries a low mortality but high morbidity. The physical disfigurement and restricted mobility lead to a loss of self-esteem, feelings of embarrassment, social stigmatization, and emotional distress. Individuals with disfiguring LF are viewed as poor marriage prospects because the disease interferes with sexual function.[40] The ADLA attacks last for 7 to 10 days and are extremely painful, debilitating, and costly. The number and severity of ADLA attacks can be reduced or prevented through the following measures:

- Frequently washing the affected limb with soap and water
- Using clean water, towels, and linen
- Drying skin carefully
- Wound care: medicated creams (antibiotics or antifungals)

Table 1
Recommended mass drug administration regimens

MDA Drugs	Administration Frequency	Eligible Population	Contraindications
Diethylcarbamazine and albendazole	Annually	Population at risk for LF transmission	• Coinfection with onchocerciasis and loiasis parasite • Pregnant women • Children <2 y • Severely ill
Ivermectin and albendazole	Annually	Population at risk for LF transmission Presence of onchocerciasis	• Coinfection with loiasis parasite • Pregnant women • Children <15 kg • Severely ill
Albendazole	Annual or biannual	Population at risk for LF transmission Presence of loiasis	• Pregnant women (first trimester) • Children <2 y • History of neurocysticercosis or seizures

Adapted from WHO. Guideline: alternative mass drug administration regimens to eliminate lymphatic filariasis. Available at: http://apps.who.int/iris/bitstream/handle/10665/259381/9789241550161- eng.pdf;jsessionid=595CD151A3776A6E8CA1FC4E89B59E2A?sequence=1. Accessed September 15, 2018.

- Clipping toe nails, inspecting between toes for open skin lesions
- Using comfortable footwear that protects the skin
- Compression bandages while ambulatory
- Elevation and exercise of affected limb
- Scrotal support

Supportive management during an ADLA attack includes:

- Bed rest with elevation of the affected limb
- Pain medication
- Antifungal ointments
- Oral or parenteral antibiotics if secondary infection is present[41,42]

Vector control:

- Permethrin-impregnated bed nets
- Clean water, sewage management, proper garbage disposal
- Insecticides[43]

The GPELF has made significant progress in many countries. Since its inception, GPELF has delivered 5.6 million treatments to more than 763 million people living in 61 countries between the years 2000 and 2014. It is estimated that the treatment has prevented 36 million clinical cases and saved 175 million disability-adjusted life years.[44,45] However, it is unlikely that LF will be eliminated by the target year of 2020. Countries that have achieved the highest success are those that have implemented innovative programs that have superseded barriers affecting participation.

BARRIERS TO TREATMENT

Studies show that gender relations and social hierarchy influence compliance with LF treatment. In many endemic countries, women's role and identity is contingent on their ability to marry and bear children. Women who do not participate in MDA initiatives fear that LF treatment interferes with fertility, promotes spontaneous abortion, and affects lactation. Furthermore, women are prohibited from participating because of their husbands' beliefs about the drug treatment.[46] In a study by Krentel and Wellings,[47] the man in the household participated in the antifilarial treatment, whereas the woman and children did not. Both the interviewed men and women stated that the man's health took precedence, because the family's health and wellbeing were solely dependent on the man's ability to work.

Nonparticipation in antifilarial treatment is associated with a lack of information, information misrepresentation, rumors, and myths. Individuals in endemic areas often associate LF with lymphedema and elephantiasis. However, without obvious symptoms, many do not believe they have the disease. In a study by Stanton and colleagues,[48] 11.8% of participants interviewed correctly identified the cause of their lymphedema as either being from a mosquito or a worm, whereas the remainder thought it was a spiritual problem, a curse, or sorcery. Malaria is accurately identified as a mosquito-borne illness, whereas LF is misconstrued as being caused by bathing in contaminated water, carrying heavy loads, stepping on insects, and contact with other infected individuals.[48] Drug side effects are also cited as a reason for nonadherence. Common, temporary antifilarial drug side effects include dizziness, headache, low-grade fever, nausea, and vomiting. However, the drugs are often perceived as uncovering other illness. The bad taste and degradation of tablets into powder because of transportation, storage, and climate challenges were also identified as barriers to participation.[10,48]

Health workers from outside the community or from other regions of the world live among the populace in an attempt to treat and control the devastating disease. Establishing trust with outsiders with an understanding of why they are present in communities is essential to an effective treatment and eradication plan. In a 2004 to 2011 study in Tanzania, fear of treatment was attributable to a lack of trust in international aid and a questioning of the motives behind the distribution.[49] Ideally, drug distributors live within the community, are personally participating in MDA treatment and protocol surveillance, and are knowledgeable about and connected to a public health system. Distribution directly in homes or in public places, such as markets, is most effective. However, despite local drug distributors, a lack of, or incomplete, knowledge is a major contributor to nonparticipation.[50]

FUTURE CONSIDERATIONS

Several factors will affect the global prevalence of LF in the future. A growing body of evidence suggests that climate change will influence the spread of parasitic diseases and their vectors. As global warming and its associated changes in weather patterns evolve, parasitic diseases such as LF could experience a reemergence in previously endemic areas or a spread to new geographic areas.[51,52] Furthermore, population shift to megacities and large cities is expected to continue over the next several decades. Many molecular epidemiologists warn that international trade, travel, migration, and land-use changes increase risk for transmittable diseases.[53] Filarial parasites exposed to MDA may mutate, reducing the effectiveness of drug therapy alone.[54] Although considerable progress has been made in global control of LF through MDA and morbidity management efforts, LF programs continue to face numerous challenges. To eliminate LF, these strategies will need to expand to include improved surveillance protocols, delivery strategies, vector control, and integration of newer techniques and technologies.[53,55]

REFERENCES

1. World Health Organization. Neglected tropical diseases. 2018. Available at: http://www.who.int/neglected_diseases/diseases/en/. Accessed August 15, 2018.
2. Centers for Disease Control and Prevention. Neglected tropical diseases. 2017. Available at: https://www.cdc.gov/globalhealth/ntd/resources/ntd_factsheet.pdf. Accessed September 1, 2018.
3. National Institute of Allergy and Infectious Diseases. Types of neglected tropical diseases. Available at: https://www.niaid.nih.gov/research/neglected-tropical-diseases-types. Accessed September 1, 2018.
4. Centers for Disease Control and Prevention. Lymphatic filariasis: epidemiology and risk factors. 2013. Available at: https://www.cdc.gov/parasites/lymphaticfilariasis/epi.html. Accessed September 1, 2018.
5. World Health Organization. Global program to eliminate lymphatic filariasis. 2010. Available at: http://www.searo.who.int/entity/vector_borne_tropical_diseases/tropics/lymphatic_filariasis/LFREP.pdf. Accessed August 20, 2018.
6. World Health Organization. Lymphatic filariasis: key facts. 2018. Available at: http://www.who.int/news-room/fact-sheets/detail/lymphatic-filariasis. Accessed August 20, 2018.
7. Zeldenryk LM, Gray M, Speare R, et al. The emerging story of disability associated with lymphatic filariasis: a critical review. PLoS Negl Trop Dis 2011;5(12):e1366.
8. The Carter Center. The life cycle of lymphatic filariasis. 2018. Available at: https://www.cartercenter.org/resources/pdfs/health/lf/lymphatic-filariasis-life-cycle.pdf. Accessed September 1, 2018.

9. McNulty SN, Mitreva M, Weil GJ, et al. Inter and intra-specific diversity of parasites that cause lymphatic filariasis. Infect Genet Evol 2013;14:137–46.

10. Celone M. Barriers to the elimination of lymphatic filariasis. J Glob Health 2015. Available at: https://www.ghjournal.org/barriers-to-the-elimination-of-lymphatic-filariasis-in-sub-saharan-africa/. Accessed September 1, 2018.

11. Shenoy RK, Suma TK, Cumaraswami V, et al. Lymphoscintigraphic evidence of lymph vessel dilation in the limbs of children with Brugia malayi infection. J Commun Dis 2008;40(2):91–100.

12. Shenoy RK, Bockarie MJ. Lymphatic filariasis in children: clinical features, infection burdens and prospects for elimination. Parasitology 2011;138(12):1559–68.

13. Goel TC. Lymphatic system. In: Goal TC, Goal A, editors. Lymphatic filariasis. Singapore: Springer Science + Business Media; 2016. p. 30–9.

14. Nascimbeni M, Shin E, Chiriboga L, et al. Peripheral CD4$^+$ CD8$^+$ T cells are differentiated effector memory cells with antiviral functions. Blood 2004;104:478–86.

15. Pfarr KM, Debrah AY, Specht S, et al. Filariasis and lymphedema. Parasite Immunol 2009;31(11):664–72.

16. Babu S, Nutman TB. Immunology of lymphatic filariasis. Parasite Immunol 2014; 26(8):338–46.

17. Nookal S, Sundaram S, Perumal K, et al. Impairment of tetanus-specific cellular and humoral responses following tetanus vaccination in human lymphatic filariasis. Infect Immun 2004;75(2):2598–604.

18. Bal MS, Mandal NN, Das MK, et al. Transplacental transfer of filarial antigens from Wuchereria bancrofti-infected mothers to their offspring. PLoS Negl Trop Dis 2015;137:669–73.

19. Madhusmita B, Manoranjan R, Ashok SK, et al. Maternal filarial infection influences the development of regulatory T cells in children from infancy to early childhood. PLoS Negl Trop Dis 2016;10(11):e0005144.

20. Debrah LS, Albers A, Debrah AY, et al. Single nucleotide polymorphisms in the angiogenic and lymphangiogenic pathways are associated with lymphedema caused by Wuchereria bancrofti. Hum Genomics 2017;11:26.

21. Chesnais CB, Sabbagh A, Pion SD, et al. Familial aggregation and heritability of Wuchereria bancrofti infection. J Infect Dis 2016;214(4):587–94.

22. Babu S, Nutman TB. Immunopathogenesis of lymphatic filarial disease. Semin Immunopathol 2012;24(6):847–61.

23. World Health Organization. Strengthening the assessment of lymphatic filariasis transmission and documenting the achievement of elimination. 2014. Available at: http://apps.who.int/iris/bitstream/handle/10665/246176/9789241508797-eng.pdf?sequence=1. Accessed September 1, 2018.

24. Rosenblatt JE, Reller LB, Weinstein MP. Laboratory diagnosis of infections due to blood and tissue parasites. Clin Infect Dis 2009;49(7):1103–8.

25. Rebollo MP, Bockarie MJ. Rapid diagnostics for the endgame in lymphatic filariasis elimination. Am J Trop Med Hyg 2013;89(1):3–4.

26. Gounoe-Kamkumo R, Nana-Djeunga HC, Bopda J, et al. Loss of sensitivity of immunochromatographic test (ICT) for lymphatic filariasis diagnosis in low prevalence settings: Consequence in the monitoring and evaluation procedures. BMC Infect Dis 2015;15:579.

27. Weil GJ, Curtis KC, Fakoli L, et al. Laboratory and field evaluation of a new rapid test for detecting Wuchereria bancrofti antigen in human blood. Am J Trop Med Hyg 2013;89(1):11–5.

28. Chesnais CB, Awaca-Uvon NP, Bolay FK, et al. A multi-center field study of two point of care tests for circulating Wuchereria bancrofti antigenemia in Africa. PLoS Neg Trop Dis 2017. https://doi.org/10.1371/journal.pntd.0005703.

29. Yahathugoda TC, Supali T, Ra RU, et al. A comparison of two tests for filarial antigenemia in areas in Sri Lanka and Indonesia with low-level persistence of lymphatic filariasis following mass drugs administration. Parasit Vectors 2015; 369. https://doi.org/10.1186/s13071-015-0979-y.

30. Lashmi J, Reddy MVR. Sensitivity and specificity of ELISA in detection of microfilariae. J Cont Med A Dent 2016;4(3):37–41. Available at: http://jcmad.com/allpapers/437.pdf. Accessed September 28, 2018.

31. Noordin R, Muhi J, Arifin N, et al. Duration of detection of anti-BMR1 IgG4 antibodies after mass-drug administration (MDA) in Sarawak, Malaysia. Trop Biomed 2012;29(1):191–6.

32. Shetty GS, Solanki RS, Prabhu SM, et al. Filarial dance- sonographic sign of filarial infection. Pediatr Radiol 2012;42(4):486–7.

33. Mand S, Debrah A, Klarmann U, et al. The role of ultrasonography in the differentiation of the various types of filaricele due to bancroftian filariasis. Acta Trop 2011;120(Supplement-1):S23–32.

34. Helder M, Colangelo AC, Schiavone M, et al. Giant elephantiasis and inguinoscrotal hernia. PLoS Neg Trop Dis 2017. https://doi.org/10.137/journal. Pntd. 005494.

35. Abeygunasekera AM, Sutharshan K, Balagobi B. New developments in chyluria after global programs to eliminate lymphatic filariasis. Int J Urol 2017;24:582–8.

36. Mullerpattan JB, Udwadia ZF, Udwadia FE. Tropical pulmonary eosinophilia – A review. Indian J Med Res 2013;138(3):295–302.

37. Ray S, Kundu S, Soswami M, et al. Tropical pulmonary eosinophilia misdiagnosed as miliary tuberculosis: a case report and literature review. Parasitol Int 2012; 61(2):381–4.

38. World Health Organization. Guideline: Alternative mass drug administration regimens to eliminate lymphatic filariasis. 2017. Available at: http://apps.who.int/iris/bitstream/handle/10665/259381/9789241550161-eng.pdf?sequence=1. Accessed September 15, 2018.

39. Centers for Disease Control. Parasites: loiasis. 2015. Available at: https://www.cdc.gov/parasites/loiasis/index.html. Accessed September 3, 2018.

40. Wijesinghe RS, Wickremasinghe AR. Physical, psychological, and social aspects of quality of life in filarial lymphedema patients in Colombo, Sri Lanka. Asia Pac J Public Health 2015;27(2):NP2690–701.

41. Chandrasena N, Premaratna R, Gunaratna E, et al. Morbidity management and disability prevention for lymphatic filariasis in Sri Lanka: current status and future prospects. PLoS Negl Trop Dis 2018;12(5). https://doi.org/10.1371/journal.pntd. 0006472.

42. World Health Organization. Morbidity management and disability prevention in lymphatic filariasis. 2013. Available at: http://apps.searo.who.int/pds_docs/B4990.pdf. Accessed September 18, 2018.

43. Bockarie MJ, Pedersen EM, White GB, et al. Role of vector control in the global program to eliminate lymphatic filariasis. Annu Rev Entomol 2009;54:469–87.

44. Turner HC, Bettis AA, Chu BK, et al. The health and economic benefits of the global programme to eliminate lymphatic filariasis (2000-2014). Infect Dis Poverty 2016;5(1):54.

45. World Health Organization. Global programme to eliminate lymphatic filariasis: progress report, 2015. Wkly Epidemiol Rec 2016;91(39):441–55.

46. Wynd S, Melrose WD, Durrheim DN, et al. Understanding the community impact of lymphatic filariasis: a review of the sociocultural literature. Bull World Health Organ 2007;85(6):421–500.
47. Krentel A, Wellings K. The role of gender relations in uptake of mass drug administration for lymphatic filariasis in Alor District, Indonesia. Parasit Vectors 2018;11:179.
48. Stanton M, Best A, Cliffe M, et al. Situational analysis of lymphatic filariasis morbidity in Ahanta West District of Ghana. Trop Med Int Health 2015;21(2): 236–44.
49. Parker M, Allen T. Will mass drug administration eliminate lymphatic filariasis? Evidence from northern coastal Tanzania. J Biosoc Sci 2013;45(4):517–45.
50. Titaley CR, Damayanti R, Soeharno N, et al. Assessing knowledge about lymphatic filariasis and the implementation of mass drug administration amongst drug deliverers in three districts/cities of Indonesia. Parasit Vectors 2018;11:315.
51. Wu X, Lu Y, Zhou S, et al. Impact of climate change on human infectious diseases: empirical evidence and human adaption. Environ Int 2016;86:14–23.
52. Rodo X, Pascual M, Doblas-Reyes FJ, et al. Climate change and infectious diseases: can we meet the needs for better prediction? Climatic Change 2013; 118(3):625–40.
53. Irvine MA, Reimer LJ, Mjenga SM, et al. Modeling strategies to break transmission of lymphatic filariasis - aggregation, adherence and vector competence greatly alter elimination. Parasit Vectors 2015;8:1–19.
54. Kwartenga A, Ahuno ST, Okoto FO. Killing filarial nematode parasites; role of treatment options and host immune responses. Infect Dis Poverty 2016;586. https://doi.org/10.1186/540249-016-1083-0.
55. Famakinde DO. Mosquitoes and the lymphatic filarial parasites: research trends and budding roadmaps to future disease eradication. Trop Med Infect Dis 2018; 3(1). https://doi.org/10.3390/tropicalmed301004.

Tuberculosis

Ana M. Kelly, PhD, RN

KEYWORDS

- Tuberculosis • Latent TB • Screening

KEY POINTS

- Although the incidence of tuberculosis (TB) is declining globally, the world is not on target to end TB in 2035.
- Drug-resistant TB is one of the greatest challenges facing the elimination of TB.
- In the United States, persons born outside the United States account for 70% of new TB cases.
- Nucleic acid amplification testing has greatly reduced the amount of time needed for diagnosis of TB, down to 1 to 2 days, compared with waiting 21 days for culture results.
- The shorter treatment regimen for latent TB infection with weekly isoniazid and rifabutin for 12 weeks provides treatment as effective as the traditional daily isoniazid for 6 months, but with better adherence from patients.

EPIDEMIOLOGY OF TUBERCULOSIS GLOBALLY

Since 2015, tuberculosis (TB), an infectious disease caused by the bacterium *Mycobacterium tuberculosis*, has overtaken human immunodeficiency virus (HIV)/acquired immunodeficiency syndrome (AIDS) as the leading cause of death from a single infectious agent.[1] However, TB is one of the most ancient maladies, with discoveries of acid-fast bacilli (AFB) and pulmonary lesions in Egyptian mummies and biblical references to a consumptive plague.[2] The 4 medications that are still used to cure drug-susceptible TB were discovered half a century ago, between 1952 and 1962. Even with this long history, TB continues to challenge the public health community. Sometimes the challenge is unexpected, such as the increase of TB coinfection with HIV in the 1990s. Other times the challenge is more familiar and persistent, such as the disproportionate burden of disease on the poor.[3]

Many in the global health community now believe the end of TB is within reach. Some of the data are encouraging, with a global TB treatment success rate of 83% and a declining incidence rate of 2% per year.[1] Since 1990, TB mortality has decreased by 47% and even the highest risk group, those living with HIV, has seen a 32% reduction in death since 1990.[4] Based on these encouraging trends, the World

Disclosure: The author has no funding sources and no conflicts of interest.
School of Nursing, Columbia University, 560 West 168th Street, New York, NY 10027, USA
E-mail address: ak3825@cumc.columbia.edu

Health Organization (WHO) set the goal of reducing the global TB incidence by 80% from 2015 to 2030, in line with the timeline of the United Nations' Sustainable Development Goals. Ultimately, the End TB Strategy outlines an effective end to TB by 2035 if each 5-year milestone is met.[4] Other data present a more dire picture. TB is the ninth leading cause of death globally. An estimated 10 million cases of active TB arose in 2017, with 1.3 million resulting in death.[1] The declining incidence rate will need to effectively double to 4% to 5% annually to reach each 5-year milestone.[4] These numbers should both encourage and challenge clinicians currently working with patients with TB.

EPIDEMIOLOGY OF TUBERCULOSIS IN NORTH AMERICA

Since 1993, TB rates have been declining in the United States, with a rate of 2.8 new cases per 100,000 population in 2017.[5,6] In North America, the greatest number of TB cases arise from foreign-born persons. In the United States, the rate of TB is 15 times higher among non–US-born persons.[5] In both the United States and Canada, 70% of TB cases occurred among foreign-born individuals.[6,7] The Centers for Disease Control and Prevention (CDC) provides annual surveillance data on TB. **Fig. 1** presents the 7 countries accounting for 61% of TB cases among non–US-born-persons, which has remained fairly consistent since 1986. The remaining 39% represents 139 other countries.[6] Eleven states reported rates of TB higher than the national average of 2.8 (**Table 1**). Demographic breakdown of TB cases in the United States reveals the highest rates among those 65 years of age and older (4.5 per 100,000), accounting for 25% of all cases. Although 60% of all cases occurred between the ages of 25 to 64 years, the higher rate among those 65 years of age and older indicates a need for clinicians to

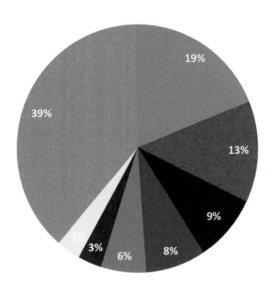

■ Mexico   ■ Philippines   ■ India   ■ Vietnam   ■ China   ■ Guatemala   ▦ Haiti   ■ Other

Fig. 1. Seven countries accounting for most new TB cases in the United States. (*Adapted from* Centers for Disease Control and Prevention, National Center for HIV/AIDS, Viral Hepatitis, STD, and TB Prevention, Division of Tuberculosis Elimination. Tuberculosis data and statistics. Reported tuberculosis in the United States, 2017. Available at: https://www.cdc.gov/tb/statistics/reports/2017/2017_Surveillance_FullReport.pdf. Accessed February 5, 2019.)

Table 1
States above the national average tuberculosis case rate of 2.8 per 100,000 accounting for 59% of cases in the United States

Rank	State	Case Rate
1	Hawaii	8.1
2	Alaska	7.2
3	California	5.2
4	District of Columbia	5.2
5	New York	4.1
6	Texas	4
7	Maryland	3.4
8	Minnesota	3.2
9	New Jersey	3.2
10	Massachusetts	3.1
11	Louisiana	3

Data from Centers for Disease Control and Prevention, National Center for HIV/AIDS, Viral Hepatitis, STD, and TB Prevention, Division of Tuberculosis Elimination. Tuberculosis data and statistics. Reported tuberculosis in the United States, 2017. Available at: https://www.cdc.gov/tb/statistics/reports/2017/2017_Surveillance_FullReport.pdf. Accessed February 5, 2019.

maintain a suspicion of reactivation of latent TB in this age group. In low-TB-burden countries such as the United States, reactivation of latent TB accounts for most new TB cases.[8] Similar to the global data provided by the WHO, TB is more common in men worldwide.[1,5] Asian people account for 36% of all TB cases in the United States. Further exploration of the data illuminates an important division: although Asians account for 49% of non–US-born patients, they only account for 5% of US-born patients. A similar trend exists with Hispanic/Latino patients, who account for 31% of non–US-born patients, but decrease to 22% of US-born patients. Combined, white people and black people/African Americans account for most US-born patients, 30% and 37% respectively.[6]

TUBERCULOSIS TRANSMISSION

TB is most commonly a disease of the lung (pulmonary TB), but can present in any organ of the body (extrapulmonary TB). Miliary TB is the term used for TB that has spread into the bloodstream. Often TB first manifests in the lungs but then spreads via the blood and lymph to other organs. Although miliary TB can lead to extrapulmonary TB, the CDC records it as a form of pulmonary TB. The most common extrapulmonary sites include lymph nodes, the pleural cavity surrounding the lungs, bones and joints, and the central nervous system (ie, meningitis). Estimates suggest 10% to 25% of TB infections are extrapulmonary, with most cases found in patients with HIV or children. Even in those more susceptible groups, patients often present simultaneously with pulmonary TB.[9] In 2017, the CDC reported 1887 cases of extrapulmonary TB with no pulmonary TB. Of these, most presented in the lymph nodes (37.8%), followed by the pleura (15.6%) and bones/joints (9.2%).[6] There were no cases of laryngeal TB, which is considered particularly infectious. The CDC classifies persons with extrapulmonary TB as noninfectious unless they also have pulmonary TB, unless the person has an open abscess. All persons with extrapulmonary TB should be tested for pulmonary TB.

Pulmonary TB is transmitted via aerosolized particles ranging from 1 to 5 mm in diameter that are then inhaled.[10] Any patient with diagnosed or suspected TB should be placed on airborne isolation. The patient is placed in a negative air pressure room and all health care workers and visitors must wear a particulate respirator (N-95) mask when entering the room.[10] Any time the patient must leave the room, the patient should wear a surgical mask. In lower-resource settings where a private negative air pressure room is not available, the health care team should take advantage of natural ventilation. Windows and doors should remain open as much as possible, fans should be used to distribute air, and clinicians should sit near the fresh air source. TB is sensitive to ultraviolet (UV) radiation and institutions often place special UV lamps that give off germicidal radiation in TB units in corridors separating patient and staff areas. Lamps should be installed away from areas that may lead to skin or eye irritation.

Guinea pigs have long been used as a predictive model of TB transmission. Effective TB treatment has been shown to render the animal models rapidly noninfectious, long before the smear or culture conversion to negative.[11] Degree of infectivity varies based on initial smear and radiographic findings. Of note, children are less infectious than adults because of their inability to produce as much sputum. The CDC outlines 3 criteria for patients to be considered noninfectious: (1) 3 consecutive negative sputum smears in 8-hour to 24-hour intervals (with 1 collected early morning), (2) symptoms improved, and (3) compliant with treatment for a minimum of 2 weeks.

One of the biggest challenges related to transmission is the number of people with active infection who are not detected. Of the 10 million new cases of TB arising globally each year, the WHO estimates only 6.4 million were diagnosed and notified, leaving a gap 4.6 million active cases undetected.[1] Without treatment, the WHO estimates that a person with active, symptomatic TB will infect an average of 10 to 15 individuals over the course of a year. The US Preventive Service Task Force recommends screening for latent TB infection (LTBI) among populations with increased risk.[12] For the US population, persons of increased risk are included in **Box 1**.

DIAGNOSIS OF LATENT TUBERCULOSIS

A quarter of the world's population is estimated to be latently infected with TB. In the United States, the LTBI estimation is 13 million.[6] Initial infection rarely results in clinical manifestations. Instead, the lungs are able to heal from the microscopic lesions produced by the bacilli, with small calcifications often left behind.[9] All TB testing, whether routine or diagnostic, begins with a symptom screen. The most common symptoms are presented in **Table 2**. Clinicians should keep in mind that patients may only present with generalized symptoms such as fever, weight loss, or lack of appetite.

Traditionally, TB screening has begun with a tuberculin skin test (TST). The TST must be delivered via the Mantoux method, with proper intradermal injection of 0.1 mL of tuberculin-purified protein derivative (PPD).[13] The proper method of injection requires the bevel of the needle to be up to produce a wheal beneath the skin, ensuring the needle has not penetrated the dermis. A positive test includes palpable induration with erythema. The presence of erythema without induration is considered a negative result. Interpretation of results is presented in **Table 3**.

At present, many clinicians and researchers are recommending the use blood-based tests called interferon-gamma release assays (IGRAs) because they only require a single visit.[14] In addition, IGRAs are the preferred tests for persons who received the bacille Calmette-Guérin (BCG) vaccine in childhood. The IGRAs use a

---

Box 1

Persons with high-risk of tuberculosis infection or latent tuberculosis infection progression in United States populations

Persons living with HIV, especially with CD4 count less than 200 cells/μL

Contacts of persons with pulmonary TB

Foreign born from a country where TB disease is common (CDC includes most countries in Latin American and the Caribbean, Africa, Asia, Eastern Europe, and Russia)

Persons receiving dialysis

Persons preparing for organ or hematologic transplant

Residence in congregate setting (skilled nursing facility or correctional facility)

Homeless

Injecting drug users

Health care workers (some sources specify only health care workers caring for patients at increased risk of TB)

Persons taking immunosuppressive medication (most notably tumor necrosis factor antagonists for rheumatoid arthritis and Crohn's disease and long-term steroids)

Persons with comorbidity that weakens immune system, most notably cancer

Persons with preexisting lung condition, most notably silicosis

Elderly (≥65 years old)

Diabetics

---

different mix of peptides from the PPD, which does not lead to a false-positive result. Reports on sensitivity and specificity for all the LTBI tests have varied widely. Besides BCG cases, the CDC holds that IGRA sensitivities are similar to those for TST. Similar to the TST, IGRAs measure immune reactivity to *M tuberculosis*. Once someone has been exposed to TB, their white blood cells release interferon-gamma when mixed with antigens. The 2 IGRAs approved by the US Food and Drug Administration (FDA) were the QuantiFERON-TB Gold In-Tube (QFT-GIT) and the T-SPOT TB test (T-SPOT). The QFT-GIT and T-SPOT have been routinely reported as functionally equivalent, although T-SPOT has a lower cost. In June 2018, the QuantiFERON-TB Gold Plus (QFT-Plus) officially replaced the QFT-GIT.[15] The fourth-generation QFT-Plus claims to have increased sensitivity (true-positive rate) for LTBI, but findings between QFT-GIT and QFT-Plus seem similar.[16] Clinicians should watch for an increased positive rate in routine screening because the QFT-Plus stimulates both CD4+ and CD8+ lymphocytes.[15] As before, none of the screening tests can distinguish active TB from latent TB.

Table 2

Signs/symptoms associated with tuberculosis (2 or more indicates positive test)

- Persistent cough lasting >2–3 wk (often begins nonproductive, but progresses to producing sputum)
- Hemoptysis (coughing up blood)
- Anorexia (lack of appetite)
- Night sweats
- Pain in the chest, often pleuritic pain (pain with inspiration)
- Fatigue (or weakness)
- Fever or chills
- Unintended weight loss

Table 3
Reading tuberculin skin test results, adapted from Centers for Disease Control and Prevention guidelines

Size of Induration	Considered Positive for:
≥5 mm	Persons who are immunosuppressed, including those with HIV and organ transplants; persons with fibrotic changes on chest radiograph
≥10 mm	Recent immigrants from high-burden countries (<5 y), residents and employees of high-risk congregate settings or mycobacterium laboratory employees, injection drug users, persons exposed to adults with known infection, children <4 y old
≥15 mm	Persons with no known risk factors

DIAGNOSIS OF ACTIVE TUBERCULOSIS

Once active TB disease is suspected, a sputum sample should be collected for smear and culture analysis. The diagnosis of active TB requires 5 considerations: (1) clinical (ie, symptom screen), (2) laboratory (ie, TST, IGRA, GeneXpert, sputum smear, and/or culture results), (3) radiographic (ie, chest radiograph findings), (4) patient (ie, known risk factors), and (5) public health factors.[17] Clinicians assess for the signs and symptoms listed in **Table 2** and any patient risk factors listed in **Box 1** during the history and physical. If TB is suspected, blood tests, chest radiograph, and sputum collection are ordered. The best time for sputum collection is in the morning as soon as the patient wakes up, before brushing the teeth. If the patient has trouble producing sputum, coughing can be induced through the use of a saline nebulizer. Do not allow the patient to simply produce spit for the sample.

Traditionally, standard microscopy with a Ziehl-Neelsen smear technique has been used to stain the AFB, producing red rods when viewed under a light microscope. Current recommendations suggest the use of fluorescent microscopy, which improves sensitivity by 10%. Use of the fluorochrome staining method produces golden-orange rods when viewed under a fluorescent microscope.[9,14,18] In either case, AFB results should be reported within 24 hours of receipt of specimen.[19] Smear results provide (1) diagnosis of the presence of mycobacteria, although they also test positive for non-TB mycobacterium, and (2) determination of the bacterial load. Bacterial load may be classified as 1+ to 3+ (using WHO classifications) or 1+ to 4+ (using CDC classifications), with definitions ranging from rare/few, to moderate, to numerous.[18]

Once a respiratory specimen is sent for culture, the result takes a minimum of 21 days for the culture to grow, plus 4 days for specimen collection and delivery. Because cultures can take anywhere from 3 to 6 weeks to grow in high-resource settings, nucleic acid amplification testing (NAAT) is frequently used because this produces sputum results in 24 to 48 hours.[14] The NAAT system currently in use in both low-resource and high-resource settings is the GeneXpert MTB/RIF system by Cepheid, which uses point-of-care polymerase chain reaction (PCR) testing to rapidly provide results on (1) the presence of M tuberculosis and (2) resistance to rifampicin. In most settings in the United States, an NAAT test is automatically performed on all AFB smear-positive specimens. For smear-negative cases, NAAT should be performed when there is a high clinical suspicion of TB. Liquid and solid cultures should still be grown even though treatment will have already begun based on smear and NAAT results.[14] In the case of extrapulmonary TB, specimens should be taken from pleural, cerebrospinal, ascetic, or joint fluids as needed. Chest radiograph results are also analyzed during this time, looking primarily for presence of cavitation, but may also show pleural effusion. Smear-positive cases with radiographic cavitation are considered extremely infectious.

DRUG-RESISTANT TUBERCULOSIS

Each year, the WHO estimates half a million new cases of drug-resistant TB (DR-TB) arise worldwide, but only 20% of those are detected and properly treated.[1] The WHO has identified DR-TB as one of the greatest challenges to achieving the Sustainable Development Goals by 2030. Drug-resistant TB presents as symptomatically identical to drug-susceptible TB. Therefore, the patient history is often the best indicator of possible DR-TB. The most important predictors of DR-TB are presented in **Table 4**. One category of data included in this table is the list of the 10 high–DR-TB burden countries, which account for 75% of the world's DR-TB cases.

Initially, DR-TB was divided into 2 categories: multidrug-resistant TB (MDR-TB) and extensively drug-resistant TB (XDR-TB). The classification of MDR-TB is defined as resistance to both isoniazid (INH) and rifampin (RIF). With XDR-TB, the bacteria are resistant to INH and RIF plus 2 additional second-line TB medications (most often one of the aminoglycoside injectable agents and a fluoroquinolone). A classification

Table 4
Important predictors of drug-resistant tuberculosis

Risk Factors	High-risk Subcategories
Previous episodes of TB treatment	1. Known or suspected nonadherence to TB treatment 2. Past documented treatment failure or relapse 3. Known administration of single-drug regimen or inadequate dosing (ie, drug shortages)
Worsening clinical or radiographic findings while on TB therapy	1. Lack of conversion of cultures to negative during first 3 mo of treatment 2. Lack of or partial resolution of clinical symptoms during intensive phase of treatment 3. Worsening or persistent radiographic findings while on treatment
Travel/origin from country with a high prevalence of DR-TB (list of 10 countries that account for the highest percentage of the total MDR-TB global burden)	1. India (23.7%) 2. China (17.3%) 3. Russia (13%) 4. Ukraine (4.3%) 5. Pakistan (4%) 6. Philippines (3.7%) 7. Myanmar (3%) 8. Uzbekistan (2.3%) 9. Indonesia (2.3%) 10. South Africa (2.1%)
Exposure to individual with known (or highly suspected) DR-TB	1. Known household contact 2. Congregate setting with known DR-TB, such as health care facility or correctional facility

Abbreviation: MDR-TB, multidrug-resistant TB.
Data from World Health Organization. Global TB report 2018. Available at: http://www.who.int/tb/publications/global_report/en/. Accessed February 5, 2019; and Curry International Tuberculosis Center and California Department of Public Health. Drug-resistant tuberculosis: A survival guide for clinicians, third edition. 2016. Available at: http://www.currytbcenter.ucsf.edu/products/drug-resistant-tuberculosis-survival-guide-clinicians-3rd-edition. Accessed February 5, 2019.

of pre–XDR-TB was used with cases of MDR-TB that had resistance to one of the second-line medications. Most cases of DR-TB are now detected via NAAT using the GeneXpert MTB/RIF system, which specifically tests for RIF resistance. This approach has led to classification of rifampicin-resistant TB (RR-TB). All RR-TB is treated identically to MDR-TB and most epidemiologic data are presented as MDR-TB/RR-TB and pre–XDR-TB/XDR-TB.[1]

A common misconception is that the primary cause of DR-TB is the progression of drug-susceptible disease caused by patient nonadherence. This theory was tested in South Africa using clinical and genotypic case definitions to calculate the proportion of XDR-TB cases caused by inadequate MDR-TB treatment (ie, acquired resistance) versus those caused by transmission (ie, transmitted resistance). Of 404 participants, 69% had never received treatment of MDR-TB and 84% belonged to one of 31 genotype clusters. These data suggested that most XDR-TB was transmitted directly between individuals as opposed to developing from patient nonadherence to treatment.[20]

As of 2018, the treatment regimen for DR-TB has been shortened and a fully oral regimen is now available. With the approval of bedaquiline and delamanid, two new medications are now available for DR-TB treatment, which has allowed the replacement of daily intramuscular aminoglycoside injections. Even with these advances, treatment of DR-TB remains long, with more side effects and worse outcomes than drug-susceptible TB.[21]

TUBERCULOSIS VACCINE

The only TB vaccine currently available is the BCG vaccine, which has been used in high-burden countries since 1921. The efficacy of BCG has been under debate since the vaccine first became available, but a large-scale meta-analysis in *JAMA* found a significant reduction in TB by 50% with the use of BCG.[22] As of September 2018, GlaxoSmithKline and Aeras are trialing a new vaccine for the prevention of active TB disease among persons with LTBI diagnosed by IGRA.[23] The phase II clinical trial is being conducted in sub-Saharan Africa among persons without HIV coinfection. After 2 years of follow-up, the incidence of developing active pulmonary TB was 0.3 per 100 persons in the treatment group compared with 0.6 in the placebo group, indicating a vaccine efficacy of 54%. Although a promising start, this vaccine must still undergo phase III clinical trials before approval.

TREATMENT OF LATENT TUBERCULOSIS INFECTION

Screening and treatment of LTBI in North America is considered crucial to controlling TB. Although only 5% to 10% of persons with LTBI progress to active TB, in the United States, the CDC estimates this could equate to 650,000 to 1.3 million cases.[24,25] The risk of developing active disease is highest in the first 2 years after latent infection.[26] The term remote TB has been used to denote old TB infection or an infection that has been adequately controlled by the immune system, but this term has not been well defined. There are 4 options for treating LTBI.[27] The options are: (1) isoniazid (INH) plus rifapentine (RPT) weekly for 3 months, (2) RIF daily for 4 months, (3) INH daily or twice weekly for 9 months, or (4) INH daily or twice weekly for 6 months.[27]

Since 2011, the CDC has recommended the shorter-course LTBI treatment regimen of once-weekly INH and RPT for 12 weeks, known as 3HP.[28] Rifapentine is a rifamycin derivative with a half-life in serum of 10 to 15 hours compared with 2 to 3 hours for rifampicin.[29] The 3HP regimen has been shown to be as safe and

Table 5
Most effective drug regimen and dosing for drug-susceptible tuberculosis

Drug	Available Drug Preparations and Safety	Intensive Phase (First 2 mo)	Continuation Phase (Additional 4–7 mo)	Adverse Effects	Patient Instructions
INH	50-mg, 100-mg, and 300-mg tablets, 50-mg/5-mL elixir, 100-mg/mL IV or IM solution Safe during pregnancy and breastfeeding (up to 20% of infant therapeutic dose is passed to baby in the breast milk)	5 mg/kg (typically 300 mg) 7 d/wk for 8 wk (56 doses total) or 5 d/wk for 5 d/wk for 8 wk (40 doses total) Pediatric dosing: 10–15 mg/kg up to 300 mg	Continue dose and interval for minimum of 18 wk (126 total doses for 7-d regimen) or 90 total doses for 5-d regimen Patients with cavitation on initial radiograph and positive cultures at completion of 2 mo therapy should receive a 7-mo (31-wk) continuation phase	Hepatitis (most age related, may exacerbate liver failure) Peripheral neuropathy (administer with 25–50 mg of pyridoxine (vitamin B6) to prevent, up to 100 mg to treat) Hypersensitivity reactions	Best absorbed on empty stomach; 50% reduction in concentration if taken with large, fatty meal Avoid alcohol Keep all formulations at room temperature Do not take antacid within 1 h of taking med
RIF, also known as rifampicin outside the United States	150-mg and 300-mg capsules, 600-mg/vial IV solution	10 mg/kg (typically 600 mg) 7 d/wk for 8 wk (56 doses total) or 5 d/wk for 8 wk (40 doses total), PO or IV Pediatric dosing: 10–20 mg/kg PO or IV	Continue dose and interval for minimum of 18 wk (126 total doses for 7-d regimen) or (90 total doses for 5-d regimen) Patients with cavitation on initial radiograph and positive cultures at completion of 2 mo of therapy should receive a 7-mo (31-wk) continuation phase	Numerous drug interactions Orange staining of bodily fluids Rash and pruritus GI upset Hepatotoxicity Thrombocytopenia and anemia	Best taken on empty stomach because high-fat meals delay absorption; take with small amount of food if causing GI upset Normal for urine, tears and other secretions may turn orange, may stain soft contact lenses Reduces effectiveness of hormone-based birth control

(continued on next page)

Table 5
(continued)

Drug	Available Drug Preparations and Safety	Intensive Phase (First 2 mo)	Continuation Phase (Additional 4–7 mo)	Adverse Effects	Patient Instructions
PZA	500-mg scored tablet	25 mg/kg/d (range 20–30) Pediatric dosing: 35 mg/kg/d (range 30–40), neither to exceed 2 g/day	Discontinue PZA for continuation phase	Hyperuricemia and arthralgia, Rash, and Hepatotoxicity Risk of toxicity with renal failure (administer max of 3 d/wk)	Report new onset of joint pain
EMB	100-mg tablets and 400-mg scored tablets Safe during pregnancy and breastfeeding	Pediatric dosing: 15–25 mg/kg/d, neither to exceed 1g/day, higher doses used during initial 2 months, doses closer to 15 mg/kg/d used to avoid toxicity	Discontinue EMB for continuation phase	Optic neuritis Risk of toxicity with renal failure (administer max of 3 d/wk)	Report any changes in vision immediately

Abbreviations: GI, gastrointestinal; IM, intramuscular; IV, intravenous; max, maximum; med, medication; PO, by mouth.

Data from Nahid P, Dorman SE, Alipanah N, et al. Official American Thoracic Society/Centers for Disease Control and Prevention/Infectious Diseases Society of America clinical practice guidelines: treatment of drug-susceptible tuberculosis. Clin Infect Dis 2016;63(7):e147–95; and Curry International Tuberculosis Center and California Department of Public Health. Drug-resistant tuberculosis: a survival guide for clinicians, third edition. 2016. Available at: http://www.currytbcenter.ucsf.edu/products/drug-resistant-tuberculosis-survival-guide-clinicians-3rd-edition. Accessed February 5, 2019.

efficacious as the longer 6HR regimen, but with substantially higher treatment completion rates. In addition, the 3HP regimen has been approved for all persons with (1) LTBI 2 years and older and (2) HIV infection, including AIDS and those taking antiretroviral therapy. Treatment may be delivered through directly observed therapy or via self-administration.[30] The CDC also recommends the use of 4 months of RIF, primarily for persons who may not be able to tolerate INH. Even after LTBI treatment, studies have shown that most patients' subsequent TB screening tests remain positive.[31] Because persons who test positive for LTBI are asymptomatic, it can be challenging for patients to initiate and remain on prophylactic treatment, especially if they experience side effects with treatment. With this list of 4 options, clinicians are able to make the best choice for their patients.

TREATMENT OF ACTIVE TUBERCULOSIS

Once active TB disease has been identified from a symptom screen, positive TST or IGRA result, and positive chest radiograph findings, the patient must be placed on treatment immediately. The 4-drug regimen of INH, RIF, pyrazinamide (PZA), and ethambutol (EMB) continues to be the regimen of choice for all cases of drug-susceptible TB. Pyridoxine (vitamin B_6) is typically given to all persons taking INH to prevent neuropathy, but at a minimum should be administered to those at highest risk of developing neuropathy, including persons with HIV, renal failure, or diabetes; persons with alcoholism or malnutrition; pregnant women or breastfeeding infants; and those of advanced age. All patients begin by taking all 4 medications every day for 2 months. Mild to moderate adverse effects are common, but serious adverse effects, such as drug-induced hepatoxicity, are rare.[32] All patients taking INH should receive baseline liver function tests (ie, alanine aminotransferase, aspartate aminotransferase). The most effective regimen for treating drug-susceptible TB is presented in **Table 5**.[17,18]

In some cases, surgical intervention is necessary. Ideally, the patient has already achieved smear conversion. Cases that are commonly referred for surgery include those in which culture remains positive after 4 to 6 months of treatment. It is more common with DR-TB, because drug-susceptible cases of TB that remain culture positive often need to first be evaluated for drug resistance. The determination to attempt a lung resection often rests on the degree and clarity of cavitation on the radiograph. After surgery, the patient must continue the medical treatment to completion.[18]

LEGAL ISSUES RELATED TO TUBERCULOSIS

Because active TB infection presents a danger to the public health, most states in the United States have enacted disease control measures. Each state has its own mandatory reporting laws, but the CDC provides a list of national notifiable infectious diseases, on which TB is included. States then provide information to the CDC voluntarily. States with a higher burden of TB, such as New York and California, have legal provisions for detaining patients who test positive for TB but refuse treatment.

SUMMARY

Although the incidence of TB is declining globally, clinicians must still maintain a high index of suspicion for TB to reach the WHO's goal to effectively end TB by 2035.[3,33]

REFERENCES

1. World Health Organization. Global TB report 2018. Available at: http://www.who.int/tb/publications/global_report/en/. Accessed February 5, 2019.
2. Daniel VS, Daniel TM. Old Testament biblical references to tuberculosis. Clin Infect Dis 1999;29(6):1557–8.
3. Gandy M, Zumla A. The resurgence of disease: social and historical perspectives on the 'new' tuberculosis. Soc Sci Med 2002;55:385–96.
4. World Health Organization. The end TB strategy. 2015. Available at: https://www.who.int/tb/End_TB_brochure.pdf. Accessed February 5, 2019.
5. Stewart RJ, Tsang CA, Pratt RH, et al. Tuberculosis – United States, 2017. MMWR Morb Mortal Wkly Rep 2018;67(11). Available at: https://www.cdc.gov/mmwr/volumes/67/wr/mm6711a2.htm. Accessed February 5, 2019.
6. Centers for Disease Control and Prevention, National Center for HIV/AIDS, Viral Hepatitis, STD, and TB Prevention, Division of Tuberculosis Elimination. Tuberculosis data and statistics. Reported tuberculosis in the United States, 2017. Available at: https://www.cdc.gov/tb/statistics/reports/2017/2017_Surveillance_FullReport.pdf. Accessed February 5, 2019.
7. Government of Canada. Surveillance of tuberculosis (TB). Available at: https://www.canada.ca/en/public-health/services/diseases/tuberculosis-tb/surveillance-tuberculosis-tb.html. Accessed February 5, 2019.
8. Getahun H, Matteelli A, Chaisson RE, et al. Latent Mycobacterium tuberculosis infection. N Engl J Med 2015;372:2127–35.
9. Heyman DL. Control of communicable diseases manual. 19th edition. Washington, DC: American Public Health Association; 2008.
10. Jensen PA, Lambert LA, Lademarco MF, et al. Guidelines for preventing the transmission of Mycobacterium tuberculosis in health-care settings, 2005. MMWR Recomm Rep 2005;54:1.
11. Dharmadhikari AS, Mphahlele M, Venter K, et al. Rapid impact of effective treatment on transmission of multidrug-resistant tuberculosis. Int J Tuberc Lung Dis 2014;18(9):1019–25.
12. Kahwati LC, Feltner C, Halpern M, et al. Primary care screening and treatment for latent tuberculosis infection in adults. Evidence report and systematic review for the US Preventative Services Task Force. JAMA 2016;316(9):970–83.
13. Mazurek GH, Jereb J, Vernon A, et al. Updated guidelines for using interferon gamma release assays to detect mycobacterium tuberculosis infection –- United States, 2010. MMWR Recomm Rep 2010;59(RR05):1–25.
14. Lewinsohn DM, Leonard MK, LoBue PA, et al. Official American Thoracic Society/Infectious Diseases Society of America/Centers for Disease Control and Prevention clinical practice guidelines: diagnosis of tuberculosis in adults and children. Clin Infect Dis 2017;64:e1–33.
15. Hogan CA, Tien S, Pai M, et al. Higher positivity rate with fourth-generation QuantiFERON-TB Gold Plus assay in low-risk US health care workers. J Clin Microbiol 2019;2(57). e01688-18.
16. Theel ES, Hilgart H, Breen-Lyles M, et al. Comparison of the QuantiFERON-TB Gold Plus and QuantiFERON-TB Gold In-Tube interferon gamma release assays in patients at risk for tuberculosis and in health care workers. J Clin Microbiol 2018;56(7):e00614–8.
17. Nahid P, Dorman SE, Alipanah N, et al. Official American Thoracic Society/Centers for Disease Control and Prevention/Infectious Diseases Society of America

clinical practice guidelines: treatment of drug-susceptible tuberculosis. Clin Infect Dis 2016;63(7):e147–95.

18. Curry International Tuberculosis Center and California Department of Public Health. Drug-resistant tuberculosis: a survival guide for clinicians, third edition 2016. Available at: http://www.currytbcenter.ucsf.edu/products/drug-resistant-tuberculosis-survival-guide-clinicians-3rd-edition. Accessed February 5, 2019.

19. Centers for Disease Control and Prevention. National TB program objectives & performance targets for 2020. Available at: https://www.cdc.gov/tb/programs/evaluation/pdf/National_TB_Objectives_2020_Targets_20160307.pdf. Accessed February 5, 2019.

20. Shah NS, Auld SC, Brust JC, et al. Transmission of extensively drug-resistant tuberculosis in South Africa. N Engl J Med 2017;376(3):243–53.

21. Lynch JB. Multidrug-resistant tuberculosis. Med Clin North Am 2013;97:553–79.

22. Colditz GA, Brewer TF, Berkey CS, et al. Efficacy of BCG vaccine in the prevention of tuberculosis. Meta-analysis of the published literature. JAMA 1994;271(9): 698–702.

23. Van Der Meeren O, Hatherill M, Nduba V, et al. Phase 2b controlled trial of M72/ASO1E vaccine to prevent tuberculosis. N Engl J Med 2018;379:1621–34.

24. Horsburgh CR Jr. Priorities for the treatment of latent tuberculosis infection in the United States. N Engl J Med 2004;350(20):2060–7.

25. Centers for Disease Control and Prevention. Diagnosing latent TB infection and TB disease. Available at: https://www.cdc.gov/tb/topic/testing/diagnosingltbi.htm. Accessed February 5, 2019.

26. Borgdorff MW, Sebek M, Geskus RB, et al. The incubation period distribution of tuberculosis estimated with a molecular epidemiological approach. Int J Epidemiol 2011;40:964–70.

27. Centers for Disease Control and Prevention. Treatment for Latent tuberculosis infection (LTBI). Available at: https://www.cdc.gov/tb/topic/treatment/ltbi.htm. Accessed February 5, 2019.

28. Borisov AS, Morris SB, Njie GJ, et al. Update of recommendations for use of once-weekly isoniazid-rifapentine regimen to treat latent *Mycobacterium tuberculosis* infection. MMWR Morb Mortal Wkly Rep 2018;67(25):723–6.

29. Tuberculosis Trials Consortium. Rifapentine and isoniazid once a week versus rifampicin and isoniazid twice a week for treatment of drug –susceptible pulmonary tuberculosis in HIV-negative patients: a randomised clinical trial. Lancet 2002;360(9332):528–34.

30. Belknap R, Holland D, Feng P-J, et al. Self-administered versus directly observed once-weekly isoniazid and rifapentine treatment of latent tuberculosis infection: a randomized trial. Ann Intern Med 2017;167(10):689–97.

31. Pollock NR, Kashino SS, Napolitano DR, et al. Evaluation of the effect of treatment of latent tuberculosis infection on QuantiFERON-TB Gold Assay results. Infect Control Hosp Epidemiol 2009;30(4):392–5.

32. Centers for Disease Control and Prevention. Adverse events. Available at: https://www.cdc.gov/tb/topic/treatment/adverseevents.htm. Accessed February 5, 2019.

33. Kelly AM, D'Agostino JF, Andrada LV, et al. Delayed tuberculosis diagnosis and costs of contact investigations for hospital exposure: New York City, 2010 – 2014. Am J Infect Control 2017;45:483–6.

Sexually Transmitted Diseases Among US Adolescents and Young Adults

Patterns, Clinical Considerations, and Prevention

Renee E. Sieving, PhD, RN, FSAHM[a],*, Janna R. Gewirtz O'Brien, MD[b],
Melissa A. Saftner, PhD, CNM[c], Taylor A. Argo, MD[d]

KEYWORDS

- Adolescents • Young adults • Sexually transmitted diseases • Epidemiology
- Clinical practice guidelines • Prevention

KEY POINTS

- Although sexually transmitted diseases (STDs) affect individuals of all ages, they take a particularly heavy toll on young people.
- Expanded, integrated, multilevel approaches are warranted to reverse recent increases in STDs and improve sexual and reproductive health outcomes for adolescents and young adults in the United States.
- Approaches must reach beyond clinics and school classrooms; capitalize on cutting-edge, youth-friendly technologies; and change social contexts in ways that encourage young people's healthy sexual decision-making.

Although sexually transmitted diseases (STDs) affect individuals of all ages, they take a particularly heavy toll on young people. Although youth aged 15 to 24 years make up just more than one-quarter of the sexually active population, they account for half of the 20 million new STDs in the United States each year.[1] Adolescents and young

Disclosure Statement: The authors have no commercial relationships to disclose.
[a] School of Nursing and Department of Pediatrics, University of Minnesota, University of MN School of Nursing, 5-140 Weaver Densford Hall, 308 Harvard Street Southeast, Minneapolis, MN 55455, USA; [b] Division of General Pediatrics and Adolescent Health, Department of Pediatrics, University of Minnesota, 717 Delaware Street Southeast Suite 353, Minneapolis, MN 55414, USA; [c] School of Nursing, University of Minnesota, 5-140 Weaver Densford Hall, 308 Harvard Street Southeast, Minneapolis, MN 55455, USA; [d] Department of Pediatrics, Pediatric Education Office, University of Minnesota, Room M136, 1st Floor, East Building, 2450 Riverside Avenue, Minneapolis, MN 55454, USA
* Corresponding author.
E-mail address: sievi001@umn.edu

Nurs Clin N Am 54 (2019) 207–225
https://doi.org/10.1016/j.cnur.2019.02.002
0029-6465/19/© 2019 Elsevier Inc. All rights reserved.
nursing.theclinics.com

adults (AYA) bear a disproportionate share of STDs for a combination of biological, behavioral, and social-contextual reasons. Variation in biological maturation; age of sexual debut; type and number of sexual partners; patterns of condom use; access to and quality of health care services, along with economic means; and educational and employment options create a confluence of factors that may protect against STDs or increase a young person's risk of contracting an STD.[1]

This article uses terms "females" and "males" in reference to biological sex, consistent with the collection of STD surveillance data, and because anatomic differences affect clinical presentations and screening recommendations. The authors recognize that this binary classification is not fully inclusive of the range of gender and sexual identities among young people.

SEXUALLY TRANSMITTED DISEASES PREVALENCE AND TRENDS AMONG ADOLESCENTS AND YOUNG ADULTS

The following section describes current rates and recent trends in common STDs among AYA, beginning with those STDs that are reportable conditions in the United States. The Centers for Disease Control and Prevention (CDC) requires reporting of chlamydia, gonorrhea, syphilis, hepatitis B and C, and human immunodeficiency virus (HIV). Herpes, trichomonas, and human papillomavirus infections are not reportable conditions.[2] This section also considers rates of pelvic inflammatory disease, a particularly severe consequence of untreated STDs among females.

This article will not cover less common STDs among AYA, such as hepatitis, chancroid and lymphogranuloma venereum. Information on prevalence, screening, and treatment for these STDs can be found in published CDC reports.[1,3]

Chlamydia

Chlamydia is the most common reportable STD in the United States. In 2017, rates of reported cases of chlamydia were highest among AYA, representing 62.6% of all cases in the United States.[1] Among females, the highest age-specific rates were among those aged 15 to 19 years (3266 cases per 100,000) and 20 to 24 years (3986 cases per 100,000). Among males, age-specific rates were highest among 20 to 24 year olds (1705 cases per 100,000).[1]

Among females aged 15 to 24 years, reported chlamydia cases increased steadily over the most recent 5-year period, from 715,931 cases in 2013 to 771,340 in 2017. A similar pattern was seen among 15 to 24 year old males, where reported cases increased from 231,506 cases in 2013 to 295,835 in 2017.[1] **Fig. 1** depicts 5-year trends in chlamydia cases among AYA by sex and age groups.

Gonorrhea

In 2017, reported cases of gonorrhea were highest among AYA, representing 44.7% of all cases in the United States.[1] Among females, the highest age-specific rates were among those aged 15 to 19 years (557 cases per 100,000) and 20 to 24 years (685 cases per 100,000). Among males, age-specific rates were highest in those aged 20 to 24 years (705 cases per 100,000).[1]

Among females aged 15 to 24, reported gonorrhea cases increased steadily over the most recent 5-year period, from 107,509 cases in 2013 to 132,151 in 2017. A similar pattern was seen among 15- to 24-year-old males, where reported cases increased from 77,267 cases in 2013 to 115,954 in 2017.[1] **Fig. 2** depicts 5-year trends in gonorrhea cases among AYA by sex and age groups.

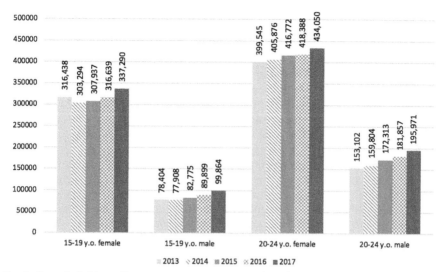

Fig. 1. Reported chlamydia cases among persons aged 15 to 24 years by age group and sex, United States, 2013 to 2017. (*Data from* Centers for Disease Control and Prevention. Sexually transmitted disease surveillance 2017. Atlanta (GA): U.S. Department of Health and Human Services; 2018.)

Syphilis

Unlike chlamydia and gonorrhea, rates of primary and secondary syphilis are substantially higher among US males than females. In 2017, syphilis rates were 3.2 cases per 100,000 15- to 19-year-old females, 7.8 cases per 100,000 20- to 24-year-old females, 10.1 cases per 100,000 15- to 19-year-old males, and 41.1 cases per 100,000 20- to

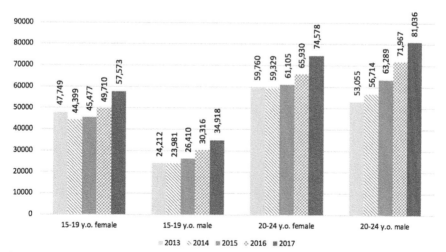

Fig. 2. Reported gonorrhea cases among persons aged 15 to 24 years by age group and sex, United States, 2013 to 2017. (*Data from* Centers for Disease Control and Prevention. Sexually transmitted disease surveillance 2017. Atlanta (GA): U.S. Department of Health and Human Services; 2018.)

24-year-old males. Males aged 20 to 24 years had the second highest rate of primary and secondary syphilis of all age groups, surpassed only by males aged 25 to 29 years.[1]

Among females aged 15 to 24 years, reported syphilis cases increased steadily over the most recent 5-year period, from 635 cases in 2013 to 1175 in 2017. A similar pattern was seen among 15- to 24-year-old males, where reported cases increased from 3904 cases in 2013 to 5820 in 2017.[1] **Fig. 3** depicts 5-year trends in syphilis cases among AYA by sex and age groups.

Human Immunodeficiency Virus

US AYA account for a substantial number of HIV infections. In 2016, the rate of HIV diagnoses was 5.8 per 100,000 among adolescents aged 13 to 19 years and 30.5 per 100,000 among young adults aged 20 to 24 years. Most new infections were attributed to male-to-male sexual contact, including 92% among male adolescents and 91% among male young adults. For females, most new infections were attributed to heterosexual contact, including 85% among adolescents and 88% among young adults. From 2011 to 2016, the rate of diagnosed infections declined among adolescents and remained stable among 20 to 24 year olds. A CDC HIV Surveillance Report details differences in AYA HIV infection, HIV, and AIDS prevalence by sex and transmission category, race/ethnicity, and region of the United States.[4]

Other Sexually Transmitted Diseases

The following paragraphs describe prevalence of STDs that are not reportable conditions in the United States.

Human papillomavirus

Human papillomavirus (HPV) is the most common STD in the United States[5]; more than 40 distinct HPV types can infect the genital tract.[6] HPV types 16 and 18 account

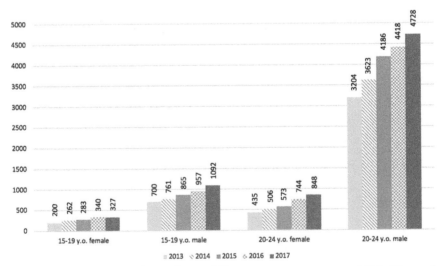

Fig. 3. Reported primary and secondary syphilis cases among persons aged 15 to 24 years by age group and sex, United States, 2013 to 2017. (*Data from* Centers for Disease Control and Prevention. Sexually transmitted disease surveillance 2017. Atlanta (GA): U.S. Department of Health and Human Services; 2018.)

for approximately 66% of cervical cancers,[7] 50% of high-grade and 25% of low-grade cervical intraepithelial lesions.[1] HPV types 6 and 11 are responsible for approximately 90% of genital warts.[1] HPV 9-valent vaccine (Gardasil 9) targets HPV types 6, 11, 16, 18, 31, 33, 45, 52, and 58; this vaccine was approved for females in 2014 and males in 2015.[8] Previously, a quadrivalent HPV vaccine targeting 4 HPV types was introduced for females in 2006 and males in 2009.[9]

Prevalence of HPV 6, 11, 16, and 18 has been estimated using data from females aged 14 to 34 years in the National Health and Nutrition Examination Survey (NHANES). Prevalence decreased significantly from the prevaccine era (2003–2006) to the early postvaccine era (2009–2012) among females aged 14 to 19 years and 20 to 24 years, age groups most likely to benefit from HPV vaccination.[10]

Herpes simplex virus

Herpes simplex virus (HSV) is among the most prevalent STDs.[5] Most genital HSV infections in the United States are caused by HSV type 2 (HSV-2), whereas HSV type 1 (HSV-1) infections are typically orolabial and acquired during childhood.[11]

NHANES data show that among 14 to 19 year olds, HSV-1 seroprevalence has decreased substantially, from 39.0% during 1999 to 2004 to 30.1% during 2005 to 2010, indicating declining orolabial infection in this age group.[11] Studies have found that genital HSV-1 infections are increasing among young adults,[12] in part due to declines in orolabial HSV-1 infections, as those who lack HSV-1 antibodies at sexual debut are more susceptible to genital HSV-1 infection.[11,13] Increasingly common oral sex behavior among AYA may be another contributing factor.[11] The absence of HSV-1 antibodies also increases the likelihood of developing symptomatic disease from newly acquired genital HSV-2 infection.[14] Thus, young women may be increasingly likely to first acquire HSV-1 infection genitally and/or to acquire a primary genital HSV-2 infection during their childbearing years.[13] First-episode HSV infection during pregnancy increases the risk of neonatal HSV transmission.[13]

Trichomonas

Trichomonas is a protozoal infection. Limited trend data suggest stable rates of this STD among persons seeking health care services.[1]

Pelvic Inflammatory Disease

Consequences of STDs are particularly severe for young women. If untreated, chlamydia and gonorrhea may ascend to the upper reproductive tract, resulting in pelvic inflammatory disease (PID), causing inflammation and damage to the fallopian tubes, increasing the risk of infertility and ectopic pregnancy. Prospective studies suggest that about 15% of untreated chlamydial infections progress to clinically diagnosed PID; the risk with untreated gonococcal infection may be even higher.[15] Recent studies suggest that the proportion of PID cases attributable to chlamydia or gonorrhea is declining; of females who received a diagnosis of acute PID, less than 50% test positive for one of these organisms.[3,16]

Accurate estimates of PID are difficult to obtain, in part because definitive diagnosis of this condition can be complex. Research suggests overall declining rates PID diagnoses in both hospital and ambulatory settings.[15] Several factors may contribute to declining PID rates, including increases in chlamydia and gonorrhea screening, more sensitive diagnostic technologies, and availability of single-dose therapies that increase adherence to treatment.[17] Although rates are declining, PID continues to cause an excessive amount of unnecessary morbidity.

SEXUALLY TRANSMITTED DISEASES TREATMENT OVERVIEW: COMMON CLINICAL PRESENTATIONS, SCREENING, AND MANAGEMENT

The following section provides an overview of key clinical features, screening recommendations, and management strategies for common STDs among AYA. First, the authors review nonviral STDs, including chlamydia, gonorrhea, pelvic inflammatory disease, trichomonas, and syphilis. They also discuss 3 viral STDs: HPV, HSV, and HIV.

The screening and treatment recommendations published by the US Preventive Services Task Force,[18] the CDC,[3] the American Academy of Pediatrics,[19] the American College of Obstetricians and Gynecologists,[20,21] and the American Academy of Family Physicians are summarized in this article.[22]

Nonviral Sexually Transmitted Diseases

Chlamydia trachomatis
Clinical presentation Most chlamydia infections are asymptomatic, with only 10% of males and 5% to 30% of females developing symptoms, highlighting the critical role of screening asymptomatic individuals.[23] Chlamydia symptoms can include cervicitis, urethritis, proctitis, and rarely pharyngitis.[19] Complications include PID, tubal-factor infertility, ectopic pregnancy, chronic pelvic pain, increased HIV transmission, adverse pregnancy and neonatal outcomes, epididymitis, and reactive arthritis.[19]

Screening and diagnostic considerations Screening and diagnostic considerations are summarized in **Table 1**. In addition to recommendations in **Table 1**, persons who have had sex with chlamydia-infected individuals during the 60 days before diagnosis should be tested and treated due to the high likelihood of infection.[3,19]

Treatment Treatment recommendations are summarized in **Table 2**. Testing for reinfection is recommended at 3 months or later within a 12-month period following infection. Test-of-cure is not needed, except in rare cases, including pregnancy or second-line treatment. It is important to note that in treating chlamydia, gonococcal coverage is not required.[3]

Neisseria gonorrhea
Clinical presentation For males, most gonorrhea infections are symptomatic; whereas for females, up to 95% may be asymptomatic. Gonorrhea symptoms can include cervicitis, urethritis, proctitis, pharyngitis, and rarely conjunctivitis. Vaginal and penile discharge is frequently mucopurulent. Complications include PID, ectopic pregnancy, infertility, adverse pregnancy and neonatal outcomes, chronic pelvic pain, epididymitis, and rarely disseminated gonococcal infection.[24]

Screening and diagnostic considerations In addition to these recommendations, persons who have had sex with gonorrhea-infected individuals during the 60 days before diagnosis should be tested and treated due to the high likelihood of infection (see **Table 1**).[3]

Treatment Gonorrhea treatment is complicated by increasing antimicrobial resistance (see **Table 2**). Cases of suspected treatment failure should be reported to local or state health departments and should prompt retesting, preferably with NAAT, culture, and susceptibilities. Testing for reinfection is recommended at 3 months or later within the 12-month period following infection, at the anatomic site of the prior infection. Test-of-cure is only required during pregnancy and for pharyngeal gonorrhea treated with an alternative regimen.[3,24]

Table 1
STD screening recommendations for adolescents and young adults

	Female		Male	
	Screening	Diagnostic Testing	Screening	Diagnostic Testing
Chlamydia	Annual screening if sexually active[a-d]	Nucleic Acid Amplification Tests (NAAT) *First choice:* vaginal swab[g]; first void urine also acceptable[a-d]	*Average risk:* insufficient evidence for screening[d] *High-risk settings[e] or groups[f]:* screen at least annually, depending on risk *MSM:* screen annually for penile & rectal infection	NAAT *First choice:* first void urine[a,c,d] *MSM:* urine and rectal[a,c,d]
Gonorrhea	Annual screening if sexually active[a-d]	NAAT *First choice:* vaginal swab[g]; first void urine also acceptable[a-d]	*Average risk:* no screening[d] *High-risk settings[e] or groups[f]:* screen at least annually, depending on risk behaviors	NAAT *First choice:* first void urine[a,c,d] *MSM:* also consider rectal and oropharyngeal swabs[c]
Trichomonas	*Average risk:* no screening *High-risk settings[e] or groups[f]:* consider screening *HIV-infected females:* screen annually[a,c]	NAAT, rapid point-of-care testing, specific culture *First choice:* first void urine or vaginal swab[g] Wet mount of vaginal fluids; sensitivity is poor (51%–65%)[a,c]	No formal recommendations	Rapid point-of-care testing, NAAT (not licensed, but may be done), specific culture *First choice:* first void urine[a,c] or meatal swabs (may be more sensitive, but less tolerable)
Syphilis	*Average risk:* no screening *High-risk settings[e] or groups[f]:* screen annually *Pregnancy:* screen at first prenatal visit; consider retesting later in pregnancy depending on risk[a-d]	Requires use of 2 tests: 1. Treponemal test: Treponema pallidum particle agglutination, enzyme immunoassay, or chemiluminescent immunoassay 2. Nontreponemal test: rapid plasma regain (RPR) or VDRL test[a-d] Often, diagnostic testing is completed using a staged approach[a-d]	*Average risk:* no screening. *High-risk settings[e] or groups[f]:* screen annually *MSM:* screen at least annually, depending on risk behaviors[a-d]	Requires use of 2 tests: 1. Treponemal test: T. pallidum particle agglutination, enzyme immunoassay, or chemiluminescent immunoassay 2. Nontreponemal test: RPR or VDRL test[a-d] Often, diagnostic testing is completed using a staged approach[a-d]

(continued on next page)

Table 1
(continued)

	Female		Male	
	Screening	**Diagnostic Testing**	**Screening**	**Diagnostic Testing**
HSV	*Average risk*: no screening. *High-risk groups*[f]: consider serologic testing[c,d]	NAAT for active lesions[a,c]. Consider type-specific HSV serologic testing for high-risk groups[f,h]	*Average risk*: no screening. *High risk*: consider serologic testing[c,d]	NAAT for active lesions[a,c]. Consider type-specific HSV serologic testing for high-risk groups[f,h]
HPV	<21 y: no screening. 21–29 y: screen with pap smear every 3 y[b,c]	Clinical diagnosis. In some instances, visual warts are tested for HPV type[c]	No screening	Clinical diagnosis. In some instances, visual warts are tested for HPV type[c]
HIV	*Average risk*: screen at least once[c,d]. *High-risk groups*[f]: screen at least annually, depending on risk behaviors[a-d]. Screening must be voluntary and free of coercion. Opt-out HIV screening is recommended, without need for specific signed consent[d]. *Diagnostic testing*: preferred tests include antigen/antibody combination tests. Rapid HIV testing can be considered; however, rapid antibody assays have a greater likelihood of false-negative results, especially in recently infected persons[a,d]			

Abbreviation: VDRL, venereal disease research laboratory.

a American Academy of Pediatrics.[19,25]

b American College of Obstetricians & Gynecologists.[21]

c Centers for Disease Control and Prevention.[3]

d US Preventive Services Task Force.[18,55–57]

e As defined by AAP, AACOG, CDC, and USPSTF, high-risk settings include jails and juvenile detention centers, national job training programs, school-based health centers, and adolescent clinics.

f As defined by AAP, AACOG, CDC, and USPSTF, high-risk groups include men who have sex with men (MSM), history of multiple or anonymous sex partners (or having sex with partners who participate in these activities), sex in conjunction with illicit drug use, sexual partners who are HIV infected, sex workers, IV drug users and who have history of sexually transmitted infections.

g Either collected by provider or self-collected, which has been shown to be highly effective and acceptable to youth.[3]

h Nearly all cases of HSV-2 are sexually acquired, so positive HSV-2 serology testing implies likely anogenital infection.[3]

Table 2		
STD treatment recommendations, adolescents and young adults[a]		
	First-Line Treatment (Outpatient Settings)	**Additional Clinical Considerations**
Chlamydia	Azithromycin, 1 g PO, single dose *OR* doxycycline, 100 mg, PO BID x7 days	Abstain from sexual intercourse for 7 d following treatment Test for reinfection in 3 mo Provide expedited partner therapy
Gonorrhea	Ceftriaxone, 250 mg, IM, single dose *PLUS* azithromycin, 1 g, PO, single dose (provides double coverage in setting of emerging resistance and treats coinfection with chlamydia trachomatis)	Abstain from sexual intercourse for 7 d following treatment Test for reinfection in 3 mo Provide expedited partner therapy
PID	Ceftriaxone, 250 mg, IM single dose (or cefoxitin, 2 g, IM, single dose with probenecid, 1 g, PO) PLUS doxycycline, 100 mg, PO BID x14 d +/− metronidazole, 500 mg, PO BID x 14 d May require parenteral therapy in more severe cases[b]	Abstain from sexual intercourse until treatment completed and symptoms resolved
Trichomonas	Metronidazole, 2 g, PO, single dose *OR* tinidazole, 2 g, PO, single dose	Avoid alcohol use during treatment
Syphilis	Parenteral penicillin G	Formulation, dosing, and duration depend on stage of disease and clinical manifestations
HSV	Acyclovir, valacyclovir, or famciclovir	Frequency, dosing, and duration depend on clinical situation (first episode, episodic, or suppressive treatment)
HPV	Provider-applied: cryotherapy (for external, vaginal, cervical, anal, or urethral), surgical removal (for external, vaginal, cervical, anal, or urethral), trichloroacetic or bichloroacetic acid (for external, anal, or cervical) Patient-applied: imiquimod, podofilox, sinecatechins (for external warts)	Observation is also an option, because many will resolve by 1 y (vs. resolution by 3 mo with topical treatments)
HIV	Antiretrovirals	Requires comprehensive care in facility with expertise in caring for patients with HIV

[a] For additional treatment options (ie, special considerations, allergies), consult CDC 2015 STD Treatment Guidelines.[3]
[b] For parenteral therapy options, consult CDC 2015 STD Treatment Guidelines.[3]
  Data from Workowski KA, Bolan GA. Sexually transmitted diseases treatment guidelines, 2015. MMWR Recomm Rep 2015;64(RR-03):1–137.

Pelvic inflammatory disease
Clinical presentation PID can present with a wide range of nonspecific symptoms that are frequently subtle. Common symptoms include abnormal bleeding, abdominal pain, dyspareunia, and vaginal discharge. Unfortunately, delay in diagnosis can result

in long-term sequelae of the upper reproductive tract, as well as progression to more severe illness. Health care providers should maintain a low threshold for diagnosis for PID.[3]

Diagnosis Presumptive treatment for PID should be initiated in sexually active females if the following 3 criteria are met:[3]

1. Experiencing pelvic or lower abdominal pain
2. No other cause for symptoms other than PID can be identified
3. One or more of the following are present on pelvic examination: cervical motion tenderness, uterine tenderness, or adnexal tenderness

Additional features that support a diagnosis of PID include an oral temperature greater than 101 F (38.3 C), cervical mucopurulent discharge or friability, abundant white blood cells on saline microscopy of vaginal fluid, elevated inflammatory markers (C-reactive protein and/or erythrocyte sedimentation rate), and laboratory documentation of gonorrhea or chlamydia infection. Although a woman with PID may have none of these features, their presence adds strength to the diagnosis.[3]

There is no specific single test for PID, and this underscores the importance of doing a pelvic examination in AYA with STD symptoms or who have suspected symptomatic gonorrhea or chlamydia.[3]

Treatment Treatment requires broad spectrum antibiotic coverage that is effective against chlamydia and gonorrhea, because negative lower tract testing does not rule out upper tract infections (see **Table 2**). Treatment should be initiated as soon as the presumptive diagnosis has been made. Although most PID cases can be treated in the outpatient setting, hospitalization should be considered for tuboovarian abscess, pregnancy, severe illness, high fever, inability to tolerate or failure to respond to oral therapy, or concern for alternative surgical emergency (ie, appendicitis). To minimize transmission and reinfection, females should abstain from sexual intercourse until treatment is completed, symptoms have resolved, and partners have been treated. All females diagnosed with chlamydial or gonococcal PID should be tested for reinfection 3 months or later within and 12-month period following PID diagnosis.[3]

Syphilis
Clinical presentation Syphilis is a systemic STD that progresses through 3 stages (**Table 3**). Feared complications include progression to later stages of syphilis, neurosyphilis, and congenital syphilis in infants of affected mothers.[3,25]

Screening and diagnostic considerations Screening and diagnostic considerations are summarized in **Table 1**.

Treatment Frequency and duration of Penicillin treatment depends on stage of illness. Laboratory response to treatment is monitored over a period of months (see **Table 2**).[3]

Trichomoniasis vaginalis
Clinical presentation Trichomonas is frequently asymptomatic, with 70% to 85% of cases with minimal or no symptoms. Symptoms can include urethritis, epididymitis and prostatitis in males. Females may experience copious, malodorous yellow-green vaginal discharge with or without vulvar irritation. Complications include increased risk of HIV transmission, increased risk of PID, and adverse pregnancy outcomes.[3,19]

Screening and diagnostic considerations Screening and diagnostic considerations are summarized in **Table 1**.

Table 3
Syphilis clinical presentations

Stage	Time	Manifestations
Primary	Starts 10–90 d after exposure; lasts several wk	Chancre (painless, indurated ulcer at the site of inoculation; heals spontaneously)
Secondary	Starts at 1–2 mo; lasts 3–12 wk	Fever, fatigue, sore throat, myalgia, arthralgia, lymphadenopathy, condylomata lata (hypertropic popular lesions affecting moist areas around vulva or anus), polymorphous maculopapular rash (palms and soles)
Latent	Early, <1 y Late, >1 y	Asymptomatic, but may be interrupted during the first few years by recurrent symptoms of secondary syphilis[a]
Tertiary	15–30 y after the initial infection	Cardiovascular syphilis (aortitis), gummatous syphilis (soft, noncancerous, but destructive growths) Neurosyphilis (CNS involvement that can occur at any stage): meningitis, uveitis, seizures, optic atrophy, dementia, posterior spinal cord degeneration

Abbreviation: CNS, central nervous system.
[a] If unknown duration, assume late latent syphilis.
Data from Workowski KA, Bolan GA. Sexually transmitted diseases treatment guidelines, 2015. MMWR Recomm Rep 2015;64(RR-03):1–137.

Treatment Treatment recommendations are summarized in **Table 2**.

Viral Sexually Transmitted Diseases

Human papillomavirus
Clinical presentation Common clinical presentations of HPV are anogenital warts and cervical dysplasia. Anogenital warts can be painful and pruritic depending on their size and anatomic location. They commonly occur on the vaginal introitus, penile shaft, foreskin, or anal region.[3]

Screening and diagnostic considerations Screening and diagnostic considerations are summarized in **Table 1**.

Treatment Goals of treating HPV-associated anogenital warts include removal of the warts and amelioration of symptoms (see **Table 2**).[3]

Herpes simplex virus
Clinical presentation The classic HSV presentation is an eruption of clustered vesicles or ulcers. However, many infected persons have mild symptoms or are asymptomatic. The first clinical episode of genital herpes can be particularly severe, with a protracted course and neurologic sequelae. Most cases of genital herpes are caused by HSV-2; however, HSV-1 can also cause genital lesions. It is important to identify the specific strain when making a diagnosis, because this affects counseling regarding prognosis and management options. HSV-2 is more likely to cause recurrences and subclinical shedding.[3]

Screening and diagnostic considerations For individuals diagnosed with HSV, HIV testing is recommended (see **Table 1**).[3,22]

Treatment Systemic antiviral medications are effective in reducing clinical symptoms (see **Table 2**). They can be used for episodic treatment (first clinical episode or recurrences) or suppressive treatment (daily). For best results, persons receiving episodic therapy should initiate treatment as soon as they notice symptoms. Suppressive treatment reduces frequency, severity, and transmission. These medications do not fully eradicate the virus.[3] Counseling regarding the natural history, modes of transmission (sexual and perinatal, with asymptomatic viral shedding), and treatment options is essential.[3]

Human immunodeficiency virus

HIV begins as an acute antiretroviral infection, transitions to a chronic progressive illness that leads to slow depleting of CD4 T cells over the course of years, and culminates with severe, symptomatic immunodeficiency. Given the range of clinical presentations and complexity of treatment, this discussion is limited to several key topics for practicing providers.

Clinical presentation of acute human immunodeficiency virus It is critical for clinicians to recognize acute retroviral syndrome, because identification at this early stage of illness represents an opportunity for diagnosis and treatment. Most individuals are symptomatic with acute retroviral syndrome within the first few weeks after they become infected. Symptoms are nonspecific and include fever, malaise, lymphadenopathy, and skin rash. During this time, individuals are highly infectious; however, HIV serologic testing during this time may yield negative results. Suspicion of acute retroviral syndrome should prompt urgent assessment with HIV-1/HIV-2 antigen-antibody immunoassay or HIV RNA in conjunction with an antibody test.[3]

Screening and diagnostic considerations Screening must be voluntary and free of coercion. Opt-out HIV screening is recommended, without need for specific signed consent (see **Table 1**).[3]

Treatment HIV treatments are now highly effective; the life expectancy for individuals with HIV is near normal, when provided with early treatment (see **Table 2**). After a new HIV diagnosis, patients should be referred to a health care facility with expertise in providing comprehensive HIV treatment. Immediate evaluation is recommended when more advanced disease is suspected (eg, fever, weight loss, diarrhea, cough, shortness of breath, candidiasis).[3]

PRACTICAL CONSIDERATIONS FOR CLINICIANS

The following section reviews the literature for best practices with AYA related to communicating an STD diagnosis, STD reporting and services for sexual partners, and confidential services.

Communicating an Sexually Transmitted Diseases Diagnosis

Communicating an STD diagnosis can be a difficult task for even the most seasoned clinician. Historically, laboratory results were communicated via mail, telephone, or office visits. With the advent of electronic medical records and online portals, more patients have access to their digital records. It is possible for patients to learn of a positive diagnosis before a clinician notifying them of the result.

Patient preference for STD notification has evolved in the last decade.[26] With increased access to smartphones, transformation of electronic health records, and online patient portals patients' preferences have shifted.

Research suggests that most text messages are read, typically within 15 minutes.[27] Shultz and colleagues[28] noted that younger adult patients preferred electronic communication modalities. A recent study found that young people and females opted for text message notification more often than their older and male counterparts; those with text messaging preferences had quicker time to treatment for STDs.[29] Given that electronic communication is often preferred among AYA, it is important to offer a variety of notification methods and provide notification based on patient preference.

Giardina and colleagues[26] found that patients older than 18 years overwhelmingly support having access to their test results, both normal and abnormal, in online patient portals. However, participants in this study also believed that a clinician should communicate abnormal results verbally to the patient before online release. It is reasonable to expect that AYA will find electronic notification acceptable and in some cases preferred. However, clinicians should ensure that they note patient preference and follow-up accordingly. Health care systems should develop online notification systems to ensure that abnormal and sensitive results of STD tests are not communicated without clinician support and education.[26]

Sexually Transmitted Diseases Reporting and Services for Sexual Partners

The CDC works with approximately 3000 public health departments around the United States to collect STD surveillance data.[30] State public health departments have their own notifiable condition requirements. Ultimately, it is a clinician's responsibility to notify local health departments about reportable STDs. Therefore, clinicians should know notifiable conditions in their state of practice and understand how to report them.

When clinicians report STDs to the local health department, they must also consider the partners of persons who tested positive. Partner notification laws vary by state and diagnosis. The greatest number of state laws about partner notification and disclosure are related to HIV. In 18 states, HIV positive persons must disclose their status to their sexual partners. In addition, 44 states have criminal laws related to willfully spreading HIV.[31]

Goals of partner services include maximizing access to information, testing services, and medical treatment for the infected individual and partner to promote community health.[2] Principles guiding partner services are that these services are client-centered, accessible, available to all, confidential, and voluntary.[2] The CDC also recommends that partner services be free; evidenced-based; part of an array of integrated services; and culturally, linguistically, and developmentally appropriate.[2] *Section IV* provides information about expedited partner therapy for chlamydia and gonorrhea.

Confidentiality

Existing literature highlights the importance of confidentiality in youth health services. Young people often avoid needed sexual health services because of confidentiality concerns.[32] All 50 states and the District of Columbia allow minors (those younger than 18 years) to consent to STD diagnosis and treatment services, although 11 states require that adolescents be at least a certain age to consent.[33] In addition, 18 states allow clinicians to inform a parent that their adolescent child accessed sexual health services, although there is no requirement to inform, except in Iowa, where clinicians are required to notify parents of HIV positive results.[33] Many state minor consent laws incorporate confidentiality protections. Despite consent laws breaches in confidentiality may still occur. Parents may learn of their AYA child's health care activities via online patient portal sites, an Explanation of Benefits (EOB) from an insurance provider, or a bill from a health care system.[34]

Health care systems can promote confidentiality by incorporating clinical guidelines from professional organizations into their policies.[35–37] Health care systems can notify

AYA seeking health services about state laws and ensure they understand how their confidentiality may or may not be protected by their insurance. In addition, health care systems can protect privacy of AYA patients by setting restrictions on information parents can access via their children's online patient portals, offering AYA the opportunity to pay out of pocket for services, or referring them to Title X-funded clinics that do not send EOBs.[34]

PREVENTING STDs AMONG ADOLESCENTS AND YOUNG ADULTS

The final section of this article details best practice recommendations for STD prevention with AYA, including correct and consistent condom use; expedited partner therapy for gonorrhea and chlamydia; preexposure prophylaxis for HIV prevention; and evidence-based prevention approaches in community settings. Our goal is to aid clinicians with practical guidelines in providing care to AYA.

Condom Use

There has been a significant decline in condom use among young people over the past decade.[38] According to the national Youth Risk Behavior Survey (YRBS), adolescent females' self-reported condom use during last sexual intercourse declined from 57.4% in 2013 to 52.0% in 2015.[38] YRBS data also confirm that many adolescents are inconsistent condom users.[39] Although reasons for declines in condom use are not fully understood, concern exists that these declines may be an unintended consequence of increases in use of long-acting reversible contraception (LARC).[40] Steiner and colleagues[40] found that adolescents using LARC were less likely than those using oral contraceptive pills to also use condoms. It is possible that a main motivation for condom use among young people is backup pregnancy prevention and with highly effective contraceptive methods, youth may not perceive a need for additional pregnancy protection. As LARC uptake continues to increase among AYA, clinicians must explicitly counsel young people about the importance of using condoms plus hormonal contraception as the most effective means of preventing both STDs and pregnancy.[41]

Expedited Partner Therapy

Because a common cause of STD infection among AYA females is reinfection from untreated partners,[42] it behooves clinicians to treat both the patients and their sexual partners. To break the cycle of reinfection and mitigate rising rates of gonorrhea and chlamydia, experts have advocated for expedited partner therapy (EPT),[43] the practice of providing prescriptions or medications to a patient or to their partner without the partner undergoing a medical evaluation. It is preferable for the partner to undergo a medical examination; however, when this is not practical, EPT should be offered.[44] EPT treatment guidelines are in **Table 4**. EPT decreases reinfection rates

Table 4 Expedited partner therapy for chlamydia and gonorrhea[a]	
Chlamydia	Azithromycin, 1 g, single dose
Gonorrhea	Cefixime, 400 mg, oral, single dose *PLUS* azithromycin, 1 g, single dose

[a] For heterosexual contacts if infected individual's partner unable or unwilling to seek medical care.

Data from Workowski KA, Bolan GA. Sexually transmitted diseases treatment guidelines, 2015. MMWR Recomm Rep 2015;64(RR-03):1–137.

compared with standard partner referrals for treatment.[44] EPT is not recommended for men who have sex with men (MSM) because of high risk for coinfections and limited data evaluating efficacy of this approach with MSM.[3] Even with proven efficacy, legal, practical, and administrative barriers hinder routine use of EPT.[44] Currently EPT is legal in 42 states. The CDC provides up-to-date information on the legal status of EPT in all 50 states.[45]

HIV Preexposure Prophylaxis

Young people are the fastest growing age group of HIV positive persons.[46] AYA at highest risk of HIV infection include lesbian, gay, bisexual, and transgender youth; youth who inject drugs; and youth who are sexually exploited or involved in sex work.[47] In 2016, 21% of all newly diagnosed HIV cases in the United States were among young people aged 13 to 24 years.[4] Young people diagnosed with this chronic, life-threatening disease face complex medical, financial, and social challenges. Condom use is the pillar of HIV prevention, in addition to HIV preexposure prophylaxis (PrEP). PrEP is offered to young people who are HIV negative and at high risk for acquiring HIV. PrEP or Truvada (tenofovir/emtricitabine) is a single pill taken daily. When taken consistently, PrEP can reduce risk of HIV transmission by up to 92%.[48] Initially approved by the Food and Drug Administration in 2012 for adults at risk for HIV, PrEP has recently been approved for at-risk adolescents.[49] Therefore, it is important for clinicians who care for AYA to educate themselves about PrEP and consider how to include this HIV prevention therapy in their counseling and referral practices.[47]

Adolescents and Young Adults Sexually Transmitted Diseases Prevention: Beyond Clinic Settings

Young people access sexual health information from a variety of sources including health care providers, parents, schools, community organizations, and digital media. Parents have a substantial influence on AYA sexual values, and beliefs. Research shows that quality parent-youth communication about sexual health can result in safer sex practices among youth.[50] However, nearly one-fourth of youth report not discussing sexual topics with a parent.[50] Within the context of providing confidential services, clinicians can facilitate parent-youth communication about sexual health. For example, clinicians can help their AYA patients see potential advantages to communicating with their parents and offer to start parent-youth discussions in ways that support the young person. Clinicians can also provide parents with general anticipatory guidance about parent-youth communication and youth sexual health topics without specifically disclosing confidential information from their AYA patients.[51]

    Findings from more than 3 decades of evaluating sex education programs in a variety of school and community settings are remarkably robust. Multiple studies indicate that participating in comprehensive sexuality education is linked to declines in STD risk behaviors, including delays in first intercourse, reductions in number of sexual partners, and decreases in unprotected sex.[52] Comprehensive sexuality education programs emphasize abstinence as the safest behavior and also promote the use of condoms and other forms of contraception for young people who do have sex. Considerable evidence also demonstrates that abstinence-only sexuality education is *not* associated with prevention of STD risk behaviors.[52] Surveys on US health education practice document recent declines in adolescents' receipt of formal sexuality education.[53]

    Digital technology, including the Internet and social media, represents an important new venue for sexuality education. Smartphone ownership has become nearly universal for US young people, with 95% of teens reporting ready access to a smartphone.[54]

The anonymity offered by digital technology in searching sensitive topics makes it a likely source of sexual and reproductive health information. Although online sexual and reproductive resources are often inaccurate, sites such as Bedsider.org, StayTeen.org, and Scarleteen.com provide comprehensive, medically accurate sexual health information tailored to AYA audiences.

Ultimately, expanded, integrated, multilevel approaches are warranted to reverse recent increases in STDs and improve sexual and reproductive health outcomes for AYAs in the United States. Such approaches must reach beyond clinics and school classrooms; capitalize on cutting-edge, youth-friendly technologies; and change social contexts in ways that encourage young people's healthy sexual decision-making.

ACKNOWLEDGMENTS

The authors would like to recognize Ms Jenna Baumgartner, MS, for her excellent editorial assistance with article preparation. The writing of this article was supported with funds from the Centers for Disease Control and Prevention (U48-DP005022-05-00; Sieving, PI) and the Maternal and Child Health Bureau (T71MC000064100; Sieving, PI). The funding agencies were not involved in the preparation, review, or approval of this article.

REFERENCES

1. Centers for Disease Control and Prevention. Sexually transmitted disease surveillance 2017. Atlanta (GA): U.S. Department of Health and Human Services; 2018.
2. Centers for Disease Control and Prevention. Recommendations for partner services programs for syphilis, gonorrhea, and chlamydial infection. MMWR Recomm Rep 2008;57(Early Release):1–63.
3. Workowski KA, Bolan GA. Sexually transmitted diseases treatment guidelines, 2015. MMWR Recomm Rep 2015;64(RR-03):1–137.
4. Centers for Disease Control and Prevention. Diagnoses of HIV infection among adolescents and young adults in the United States and 6 dependent areas, 2011-2016. HIV Surveillance Supplemental Report 2018;23(3):1–45.
5. Satterwhite CL, Torrone E, Meites E, et al. Sexually transmitted infections among US women and men: prevalence and incidence estimates, 2008. Sex Transm Dis 2013;40(3):187–93.
6. de Villiers E-M, Fauquet C, Broker TR, et al. Classification of papillomaviruses. Virology 2004;324(1):17–27.
7. Saraiya M, Unger ER, Thompson TD, et al. US assessment of HPV types in cancers: implications for current and 9-Valent HPV vaccines. J Natl Cancer Inst 2015; 107(6):djv086.
8. US Food and Drug Administration. Approved products: gardasil 9 2018. Available at: https://www.fda.gov/biologicsbloodvaccines/vaccines/approvedproducts/ucm426445.htm. Accessed October 11, 2018.
9. Centers for Disease Control and Prevention. FDA licensure of quadrivalent human papillomavirus vaccine (HPV4, Gardasil) for use in males and guidance from the advisory committee on immunization practices (ACIP). MMWR Recomm Rep 2010;59(20):630–2.
10. Markowitz LE, Liu G, Hariri S, et al. Prevalence of HPV after introduction of the vaccination program in the United States. Pediatrics 2016;137(3).
11. Bradley H, Markowitz LE, Gibson T, et al. Seroprevalence of herpes simplex virus types 1 and 2—United States, 1999–2010. J Infect Dis 2014;209(3):325–33.

12. Bernstein DI, Bellamy AR, Hook EW III, et al. Epidemiology, clinical presentation, and antibody response to primary infection with herpes simplex virus type 1 and type 2 in young women. Clin Infect Dis 2013;56(3):344–51.
13. Kimberlin DW. The scarlet H. J Infect Dis 2014;209(3):315–7.
14. Langenberg AGM, Corey L, Ashley RL, et al. A prospective study of new infections with herpes simplex virus type 1 and type 2. N Engl J Med 1999;341(19): 1432–8.
15. Sutton MY, Sternberg M, Zaidi A, et al. Trends in pelvic inflammatory disease hospital discharges and ambulatory visits, United States, 1985–2001. Sex Transm Dis 2005;32(12):778–84.
16. Burnett AM, Anderson CP, Zwank MD. Laboratory-confirmed gonorrhea and/or chlamydia rates in clinically diagnosed pelvic inflammatory disease and cervicitis. Am J Emerg Med 2012;30(7):1114–7.
17. Owusu-Edusei K, Bohm MK, Chesson HW, et al. Chlamydia screening and pelvic inflammatory disease: Insights from exploratory time–series analyses. Am J Prev Med 2010;38(6):652–7.
18. US Preventive Services Task Force. Final recommendation statement: Chlamydia and gonorrhea: screening 2016. Available at: https://www.uspreventive servicestaskforce.org/Page/Document/RecommendationStatementFinal/chlamydia-and-gonorrhea-screening. Accessed September 20, 2018.
19. American Academy of Pediatrics & Society for Adolescent Health and Medicine. Screening for nonviral sexually transmitted infections in adolescents and young adults. Pediatrics 2014;134(1):e302.
20. American College of Obstetricians and Gynecologists. Committee opinion no. 645: dual therapy for gonococcal infections. Obstet Gynecol 2015;126(5):e95–9.
21. American College of Obstetricians and Gynecologists. Well-woman visit. ACOG committee opinion no. 755. Obstet Gynecol 2018;126:e95–9.
22. Lee KC, Ngo-Metzger Q, Wolff T, et al. Sexually transmitted infections: recommendations from the US Preventive Services Task Force. Am Fam Physician 2016;94(11):907–15.
23. Farley TA, Cohen DA, Elkins W. Asymptomatic sexually transmitted diseases: the case for screening. Prev Med 2003;36(4):502–9.
24. Mayor MT, Roett MA, Uduhiri KA. Diagnosis and management of gonococcal infections. Am Fam Physician 2012;15(86):931–8.
25. American Academy of Pediatrics. Red book: sections on syphilis, HIV, and HSV. 31st edition. Itasca (IL): AAP; 2018.
26. Giardina TD, Modi V, Parrish DE, et al. The patient portal and abnormal test results: an exploratory study of patient experiences. Patient Exp J 2015;2(1): 148–54.
27. McCue T. 13 SMS text messaging services for marketing in the mobile age 2016. Available at: https://smallbiztrends.com/2012/05/13-sms-text-messaging-services. html. Accessed September 21, 2018.
28. Shultz SK, Wu R, Matelski JJ, et al. Patient preferences for test result notification. J Gen Intern Med 2015;30(11):1651–6.
29. Rodriguez-Hart C, Gray I, Kampert K, et al. Just text me! Texting sexually transmitted disease clients their test results in Florida, February 2012–January 2013. Sex Transm Dis 2015;42(3):162–7.
30. Centers for Disease Control and Prevention. National notifiable diseases surveillance system (NNDSS) 2018. Available at: https://wwwn.cdc.gov/nndss/. Accessed September 20, 2018.

31. National Network to End Domestic Violence. Positively safe project: the intersection of domestic violence and HIV/AIDS. Available at: https://nnedv.org/dv-hivaids-toolkit/. Accessed October 1, 2018.

32. Copen CE, Dittus PJ, Leichliter JS. Confidentiality concerns and sexual reproductive health care among adolescents and young adults aged 15-25. Hyattsville (MD): National Center for Health Statistics; 2016.

33. Guttmacher Institute. State laws and policies: minor's access to STI services 2018. Available at: https://www.guttmacher.org/state-policy/explore/minors-access-sti-services. Accessed September 21, 2018.

34. Altarum Institute. Why screen for chlamydia? A how-to implementation guide for healthcare providers. Washington, DC: Altarum Institute; 2016.

35. Alderman EM. AMA guidelines for adolescent preventive services (GAPS): recommendations and rationale. JAMA 1994;272(12):980–1.

36. American Academy of Pediatrics. Bright futures. 3rd edition. Elk Grove Village (IL): AAP; 2007.

37. American College of Obstetricians and Gynecologists. Primary and preventive health care for female adolescents. Guidelines for Adolescent Health. Washington, DC: ACOG; 2011.

38. Harper CR, Steiner RJ, Lowry R, et al. Variability in condom use trends by sexual risk behaviors: findings from the 2003–2015 National Youth Risk Behavior Surveys. Sex Transm Dis 2018;45(6):400–5.

39. Kann L, McManus T, Harris WA, et al. Youth risk behavior surveillance - United Sates, 2015. MMWR Surveill Summ 2016;65(SS-6):1–174.

40. Steiner RJ, Liddon N, Swartzendruber AL, et al. Long-acting reversible contraception and condom use among female US high school students: Implications for sexually transmitted infection prevention. JAMA Pediatr 2016;170(5):428–34.

41. Jaccard J, Levitz N. Counseling adolescents about contraception: towards the development of an evidence-based protocol for contraceptive counselors. J Adolesc Health 2013;52(4, Suppl):S6–13.

42. Hsii A, Hillard P, Yen S, et al. Pediatric residents' knowledge, use, and comfort with expedited partner therapy for STIs. Pediatrics 2012;130(4):705–11.

43. Centers for Disease Control and Prevention. Expedited partner therapy in the management of sexually transmitted diseases. Atlanta (GA): U.S. Department of Health and Human Services; 2006.

44. American College of Obstetricians and Gynecologists. Expedited partner therapy. ACOG committee opinion no. 737. Obstet Gynecol 2018;131(6):e190–3.

45. Centers for Disease Control and Prevention. Legal status of expedited partner therapy (EPT) 2018. Available at: https://www.cdc.gov/std/ept/legal/default.htm. Accessed October 1, 2018.

46. Chenault K, Waddell J, Tepper V. Pediatric providers and HIV pre-exposure prophylaxis. Pediatrics 2018;141(1):247.

47. Leonard A, Cooper MB, Fields EL, et al. HIV pre-exposure prophylaxis medication for adolescents and young adults: a position paper of the Society for Adolescent Health and Medicine. J Adolesc Health 2018;63(4):513–6.

48. Centers for Disease Control and Prevention. Pre-exposure prophylaxis (PrEP) 2018. Available at: https://www.cdc.gov/hiv/risk/prep/index.html. Accessed October 1, 2018.

49. American Academy of Pediatrics. HIV-1 PrEP drug can be part of strategy to prevent infection in at-risk adolescents 2018. Available at: http://www.aappublications.org/news/2018/06/28/fdaupdate062818. Accessed October 1, 2018.

50. Widman L, Choukas-Bradley S, Noar SM, et al. Parent-adolescent sexual communication and adolescent safer sex behavior: a meta-analysis. JAMA Pediatr 2016; 170(1):52–61.
51. Ford CA, Davenport AF, Meier A, et al. Partnerships between parents and health care professionals to improve adolescent health. J Adolesc Health 2011;49(1): 53–7.
52. Chin HB, Sipe TA, Elder R, et al. The effectiveness of group-based comprehensive risk-reduction and abstinence education interventions to prevent or reduce the risk of adolescent pregnancy, human immunodeficiency virus, and sexually transmitted infections: two systematic reviews for the guide to community preventive services. Am J Prev Med 2012;42(3):272–94.
53. Lindberg LD, Maddow-Zimet I, Boonstra H. Changes in adolescents' receipt of sex education, 2006–2013. J Adolesc Health 2016;58(6):621–7.
54. Pew Research Center. Teens, social media & technology 2018. Available at: http://www.pewinternet.org/2018/05/31/teens-social-media-technology-2018/. Accessed October 1, 2018.
55. US Preventive Services Task Force. Final update summary: Syphilis infection in nonpregnant adults and adolescents: screening. 2016. Available at: https://www.uspreventiveservicestaskforce.org/Page/Document/UpdateSummaryFinal/syphilis-infection-in-nonpregnant-adults-and-adolescents. Accessed October 11, 2018.
56. US Preventive Services Task Force. Human immunodeficiency virus infection: screening. 2016. Available at: https://www.uspreventiveservicestaskforce.org/Page/Document/UpdateSummaryFinal/human-immunodeficiency-virus-hiv-infection-screening. Accessed October 11, 2018.
57. US Preventive Services Task Force. Genital herpes infection: serologic screening. 2018. Available at: https://www.uspreventiveservicestaskforce.org/Page/Document/UpdateSummaryFinal/genital-herpes-screening1. Accessed October 11, 2018.

Seasonal Influenza (Flu)

Linda J. Keilman, DNP, GNP-BC

KEYWORDS

- Seasonal influenza • Influenza prevention • Special populations
- Management recommendations

KEY POINTS

- Seasonal influenza (SI) is an annual respiratory virus that is highly contagious and can increase morbidity and mortality in some individuals.
- The Centers for Disease Control and Prevention announced on September 26, 2018, that during the 2017 to 2018 flu season, more than 80,000 individuals in the United States died from SI and its related complications.
- SI is preventable, with annual influenza vaccination the priority evidence-based intervention. The vaccine is readily available and, in some cases, free of cost.

INTRODUCTION

Imagine an airborne respiratory virus that is highly infectious and comes on suddenly, is continuously evolving, and attacks and kills human beings every year in the United States during the late fall through early spring. This viral illness infects the respiratory system—nose, mouth, throat, and lungs. Spread of the virus is through coughing, sneezing, talking (within 6 ft), or coming into contact with contaminated surfaces (hands, doorknobs, cell phones, and computer keypads) and then touching the eyes, nose, or mouth.[1] The virus is most contagious in the first 3 days to 4 days after symptoms begin; however, healthy individuals can infect others before they experience their own symptoms. Contagion can last from 5 days to 7 days; symptoms can hang on for up to 2 weeks or longer.[2] caregivers can have this condition many times during their lifetime.[3] The virus leads to loss of time in school, work sick days, and discomfort and, in some special populations, can lead to hospitalization and even death.[4] Those individuals most at risk for severe symptoms and complications from this virus are the very young, vulnerable older adults, pregnant women, immunocompromised individuals of all ages, and those with chronic comorbid conditions.[3] Perhaps the most interesting fact about this viral respiratory condition is that, in most cases, it is preventable. Prevention is safe and readily available. What is this contagious condition? Seasonal influenza (SI)—or the flu.

Disclosure Statement: The author (L.J. Keilman) has no disclosures or funding to report and no commercial or financial conflicts of interest.
Michigan State University, College of Nursing, 1355 Bogue Street, A126 Life Science Building, East Lansing, MI 48824-1317, USA
E-mail address: keilman@msu.edu

This article lays a foundation of understanding by describing some of the epidemiology and genetics related to the virus and delineates risk factors and symptoms. Also covered are diagnosis; management plan, including self-care education and prevention; and special populations at high risk for complications from SI.

EPIDEMIOLOGY AND GENETICS

The reproduction rate (pattern and speed by which a disease moves) and critical community size (numbers of susceptible populations) determine the prevalence (number of individuals in an affected population) and incidence (occurrence of a disease within a population over a specific time frame).[5] The incidence of SI changes every year, meaning there is no incremental protection from previous vaccinations.[6] To keep track of the current weekly US Influenza Surveillance Report, go to https://www.cdc.gov/flu/weekly/. There are 3 types of SI viruses that commonly infect humans; A, B, and C. The types of human SI viruses are listed in **Box 1**.

Influenza A SI viruses are divided into subtypes based on the variety and combinations of proteins that occur on the virus surface: the hemagglutinin protein (HA) and the neuraminidase protein (NA).[3] There are 18 different HA subtypes and 11 different NA subtypes (H1–H18 and N1–N11).[11] Influenza A also is divided into different strains: currently there are influenza A (H1N1) and influenza A (H3N2).[3] Influenza A viruses also can undergo characteristic changes in the HA and NA glycoproteins: antigenic shifts (abrupt major changes associated with epidemics and pandemics) and antigenic drifts (minor changes that happen occasionally and are associated with localized outbreaks) are common.[12,13] New influenza virus variations seem related to changes that occur during viral replication and result in antigenic drift or shift.[14] Antibodies to HA and NA decrease the likelihood of an individual developing an infection.[14]

Genetic changes occur in influenza A and influenza B viruses over time and this phenomenon changes the configuration of the phylogenetic tree (a graphic depiction of the relative differences between influenza viruses).[7] An influenza viral genome is composed of all genes that create the virus.[7] The A/B viruses are RNA with 8 gene segments. These genes contain instructions for creating new viruses. Once an individual is infected, the A/B influenza viruses use the encoded instructions to trick the cell into producing more influenza viruses that spread the infection: within the individual and to other people.[7]

Globally (every year since 1980), the Centers for Disease Control and Prevention (CDC) has been working with other public health laboratories sequencing influenza viral genes. Genome sequencing reveals the sequence of the gene nucleotides.[7]

Box 1
Types of human seasonal influenza viruses

- Influenza A and influenza B cause yearly seasonal epidemics in the United States; influenza B primarily infects humans; influenza A can infect nonhuman hosts.[7,8]
  - An epidemic is (1) a sudden increase in the number of cases of a disease above what is usually expected[5] or (2) a problem that has grown out of control.[9]
  - A new/different strain of this virus type can cause a pandemic. A pandemic (1) is when a previously noncirculated influenza virus emerges and is transmitted to humans who do not have immunity[3]; (2) has an impact on a large number of people; (3) spreads over a large geographic area[5]; and (4) has an outbreak that can occur outside of the usual influenza season.[3]
- Influenza C generally causes mild respiratory illness; is associated with sporadic cases and minor localized outbreaks; only affects humans; is not believed to cause epidemics[3]; and generally is not included in the SI vaccine[10]

Comparing the nucleotide composition in 1 virus gene with the composition of the nucleotides in a different virus gene can reveal variations. Genetic variations are important because they affect the structure of the influenza virus surface proteins composed of sequences of amino acids.[7] The substitution of 1 amino acid for another can influence how well a virus transmits between people and how susceptible the virus is to antiviral drugs or current vaccines.[7]

Through genetic sequencing research, genetic library repositories now exist so scientists can compare circulating influenza viruses with the genes of older viruses and viruses used in vaccines. Through this genetic characterization, the CDC can make informed decisions regarding

- How flu viruses are compared and evolving
- The genetic variations or substitutions/mutations that appear when viruses begin spreading more easily, causing more severe disease or developing resistance to antiviral drugs
- How well an SI vaccine might protect against a particular influenza virus
- Adaptations in influenza viruses circulating in animal populations that may enable the virus to infect humans[7]

Each sequence from a specific influenza virus has its own branch on the phylogenetic tree.[7] The degree of genetic difference (number of nucleotide differences) between viruses is represented by the length of the horizontal lines (branches) in the tree. The farther apart viruses are on the horizontal axis of a phylogenetic tree, the more genetically different the viruses are to one another. **Fig. 1** is the representation of a phylogenetic tree. Genetic characterization reveals differences in viruses. For example, over the course of a flu season, circulating viruses change genetically, causing them to become distinctly different from the corresponding vaccine virus. This is an indication that a different vaccine virus may be necessary in the next flu season. The HA and NA surface proteins of influenza viruses are antigens, which means they are recognized by the immune system and are capable of triggering an immune response, including production of antibodies that can block infection. Antigenic characterization refers to the analysis of a virus's reaction with antibodies to help assess how it relates to another virus.[7]

Fig. 2 demonstrates the different features of an influenza virus, including the surface proteins HA and NA. After influenza infection or after receiving an influenza vaccine, the body's immune system develops antibodies that recognize and bind to antigenic sites

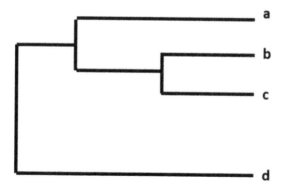

Fig. 1. Phylogenetic trees demonstrate the relationship among different flu viruses that share a common ancestor. (*Adapted from* Centers for Disease Control and Prevention. Influenza virus genome sequencing and genetic characterization. 2017. Available at: https://www.cdc.gov/flu/professionals/laboratory/genetic-characterization.htm. Accessed October 21, 2018.)

AN INFLUENZA VIRUS

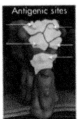

Hemagglutinin

Neuraminidase

M2 ion channel

Ribonucleoprotein

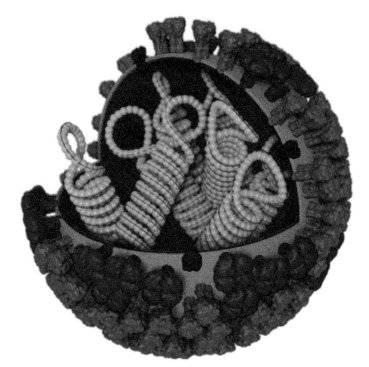

Fig. 2. Demonstrates the various features of an influenza virus, including the surface proteins HA and NA. After developing the flu or having a flu vaccine, the body's immune system develops antibodies that recognize and bind to antigenic sites or the regions found on an influenza virus's surface proteins. By binding to these antigenic sites, antibodies neutralize flu viruses, which prevents them from causing further infection. (*Adapted from* Centers for Disease Control and Prevention. Antigenic characterization. 2017. Available at: https://www.cdc.gov/flu/professionals/laboratory/antigenic.htm. Accessed October 21, 2018.)

(regions found on an influenza virus's surface proteins). By binding to these antigenic sites, antibodies neutralize flu viruses and prevent them from causing further infection.[2]

Influenza B viruses are broken down into lineages and strains.[3] At this time, there are 2 types of circulating influenza B viruses (B/Victoria and B/Yamagata), named after the geographic area where they were originally discovered.[11]

RISK FACTORS

A risk factor is any attribute, characteristic, or exposure of an individual that increases the likelihood of developing a disease.[15] Risk factor impact increases over the life course. Risk factors for contracting SI include[16]

- Age: young children and older adults (over 65 years; frail, vulnerable)
- Group conditions: being in populated environments (school, work, group home, day care, nursing facilities, military barracks, or dorms) increases exposure risk to many viruses and bacteria

- Weakened immune system: with increasing age, there are changes in the immune system that leave older adults more prone to viruses, bacteria, malignancy, and autoimmune disorders; cancer treatments; antirejection drugs; corticosteroids; and HIV/AIDS
- Long-term medication use: recent research suggests the long-term use of some medications by older adults decreases the impact of SI immunization[17]
- Chronic conditions (**Box 2**)
- Special populations: discussed later (pregnancy and obesity)

Knowing the risk factors for SI should assist health care providers (HCPs) in encouraging prevention and immunization every year. Differentiating symptoms of SI from other acute or chronic conditions is extremely important in accurate and timely diagnosis and management.

SYMPTOMS

Symptoms of influenza are unique to each individual and may present from mild to severe. Age and the presence of comorbid chronic conditions are factors in severity. Common signs and symptoms are listed in **Box 3**.

PREVENTION

The most effective and evidence-based intervention to deter SI is through yearly vaccination, as soon as it is available in the fall. Vaccinations protect human beings from preventable diseases and the burden and decreased quality of life they can cause. Continued immunization is necessary because viruses, such as SI, still exist and are constantly morphing. Eradication of diseases, like smallpox, have been possible through ongoing research and effective vaccination programs. The current recommendation is flu vaccinations at 6 months of age; there is no age end date, although vaccines for individuals over 65 have a higher potency.[10] To protect children

---

Box 2
Preexisting disease states or treatment that can lead to complications from the influenza virus

- Asthma
- Blood disorders (anemias and sickle cell disease)
- Chronic lung disease (bronchiectasis, chronic obstructive pulmonary disease, or cystic fibrosis)
- Long-term aspirin therapy (children/adolescents younger than 19 years of age)
- Endocrine disorders (diabetes)
- Heart disease (congenital, coronary heart disease, or heart failure)
- Kidney disorders
- Liver disorders
- Metabolic disorders (diabetes, inherited metabolic disorders, and mitochondrial disorders)
- Morbid obesity
- Neurologic and neurodevelopmental conditions (cerebral palsy, epilepsy, stroke, intellectual disorder, severe developmental delay, muscular dystrophy, spinal cord injury, and other disorders of the brain, peripheral nerve, spinal cord, and muscles)
- Weakened immune system due to disease or medication (AIDS, HIV, cancer, chemotherapy, or chronic steroid use)

Adapted from People at high risk of developing serious flu-related complications. Source: Centers for Disease Control and Prevention, National Center for Immunization and Respiratory Disease. Available at: https://www.cdc.gov/flu/about/disease/high_risk.htm. Accessed October 21, 2018.

Box 3
Common signs and symptoms of the flu

- Abrupt (sudden) onset
- Chills
- Cough (dry, persistent; with or without chest discomfort)
- Diaphoresis
- Discomfort (generalized)
- Fatigue (exhaustion or tiredness)
- Fever (sudden onset; if present, may last 3–4 days)
- Headache (frontal or retro-orbital)
- Myalgia (muscle/body aches; especially arms, legs, and back)
- Nasal congestion or rhinorrhea
- Pain (joints)
- Pharyngitis (sore throat)
- Sneezing
- Weakness
- In young children and frail older adults: may experience nausea/vomiting, which can lead to viral pneumonia or secondary bacterial pneumonia; diarrhea (this is not the same virus that causes vomiting and diarrhea)[18]

Adapted from CDC and American Lung Association. Lung health & diseases. 2018. Available at: https://www.lung.org/lung-health-and-diseases/lung-disease-lookup/influenza/. Accessed October 21, 2018.

---

younger than 6 months of age, parents should vaccinate themselves and keep babies safe from exposure to SI nonvaccinated individuals.[19] For helpful information on all childhood immunizations, visit https://www.cdc.gov/vaccines/vac-gen/10-shouldknow.htm.

The influenza virus is constantly evolving, which means that every year the composition of the flu vaccine is reconfigured; reconfiguration is based on the viral strains that researchers believe will potentially cause the most illness and burden. This is part of the evidence-based rationale for annual immunization. Additionally, there are self-care interventions individuals can put in place to try to stay SI-free. **Box 4** contains a summary of the interventions.

More than 200,000 individuals are hospitalized from SI complications every year in the United States. Approximately 36,000 individuals die from SI yearly.[16] If an HCP is practicing holistic, person-centered integrative care for all patients, prevention and health promotion interventions should be used prior to flu season to prevent contracting SI. Educating patients about prevention helps them recognize when they need to make an appointment with their HCP. Proactive and thoughtful decisions mutually determined with the HCP decrease complications, hospitalizations, and the overall cost of health care from an SI. Recognizing SI symptoms is paramount in timely diagnosis, treatment, and management.

DIAGNOSING

Diagnosis of SI is possible from symptoms, obtained through a holistic health history—a person's story and the HCP's clinical judgment. The person's story includes

Box 4
Self-care protective interventions to prevent influenza

- Frequent handwashing with soap and warm water for at least 30 seconds (the time it takes to sing Happy Birthday twice)[10]
- Drying hands thoroughly after washing[20]
- Keeping hands away from eyes, nose, and mouth
- Avoiding crowds and large indoor gatherings
- Covering the mouth and nose when coughing or sneezing; disposing of tissues properly
- Restful sleep
- Physical activity
- Protective barriers (wearing mask and/or gloves)[21]
- Maintaining proper nutrition
- Decreasing stress; developing positive, healthy coping strategies
- Taking time for self
- Having meaningful activities that can be done at home alone; they provide distraction, relieve tension, promote a healthy attitude, and are fun
- Keeping in touch with family, friends, and neighbors (social support) by telephone
- Staying home from work, school, and public places if not feeling well

knowledge of past medical, social, and medication histories as well as personal health and life goals. Symptoms alone are not necessarily diagnostic and can mimic other acute illnesses.[21] The HCP may need to conduct a focused physical examination. Additionally, there are diagnostic tests available to help with the decision-making process. Diagnostic testing can be helpful for special populations.

Rapid influenza diagnostic tests (RIDTs) can detect influenza viruses in respiratory specimens. RIDTs detect the viral antigens that stimulate an immune response. Rapid molecular assays detect genetic material of the virus[22] (**Table 1**). AN HCP swabs the

Table 1
Influenza virus testing methods

Method[a]	Types Detected	Acceptable Specimens[b]	Test Time	Clinical Laboratory Improvement Amendments Waived[c]
RIDTs[d] (antigen detection)	A and B	NP swab, aspirate or wash, nasal swab, aspirate or wash, throat swab	<15 min	Yes/No
Rapid molecular assay (influenza viral RNA or nucleic acid detection)	A and B	NP swab, nasal swab	15–30 min[e]	Yes/No[e]
Immunofluorescence, direct or indirect fluorescent antibody staining (antigen detection)	A and B	NP[4] swab or wash, bronchial wash, nasal or endotracheal aspirate	1–4 h	No

(continued on next page)

Table 1
(continued)

Method[a]	Types Detected	Acceptable Specimens[b]	Test Time	Clinical Laboratory Improvement Amendments Waived[c]
Reverse transcription– polymerase chain reaction[f] (singleplex and multiplex; real time and other RNA based) and other molecular assays (influenza viral RNA or nucleic acid detection)	A and B	NP swab, throat swab, NP or bronchial wash, nasal or endotracheal aspirate, sputum	Varies: 1–8 h, varies by the assay	No
Rapid cell culture (shell vials; cell mixtures; yields live virus)	A and B	NP swab, throat swab, NP or bronchial wash, nasal or endotracheal aspirate, sputum (specimens placed in VTM)	1–3 d	No
Viral tissue cell culture (conventional; yields live virus)	A and B	NP swab, throat swab, NP or bronchial wash, nasal or endotracheal aspirate, sputum (specimens placed in VTM)	3–10 d	No

Abbreviations: CLIA, Clinical Laboratory Improvement Amendments; NP, nasopharyngeal; VTM, viral transport media.

[a] Serologic (antibody detection) testing is not recommended for routine patient diagnosis and cannot inform clinical management. A single acute serum specimen for SI serology is uninterpretable and should not be collected. Serologic testing for detection of antibodies to SI viruses is useful for research studies and requires collection of appropriately timed acute and convalescent serum specimens and testing of paired sera at specialized research or public health laboratories.

[b] Approved clinical specimens vary by influenza test. Consult the manufacturer's package insert for the approved clinical specimens for each test.[38] Approved respiratory specimens vary among FDA-cleared influenza assays.

[c] CLIA of 1988. http://www.cms.gov/Regulations-and-Guidance/Legislation/CLIA/index.html.

[d] Chromatographic-based and/or fluorescence-based lateral flow and membrane-based immunoassays. Some approved RIDTs use an analyzer reader device.

[e] Rapid molecular assays can provide results in approximately 15 minutes to 30 minutes. Alere i Influenza A&B is FDA cleared for use with both nasal swabs (direct) and NP or nasal swabs in VTM and CLIA-waived for use with nasal swabs (direct) only. Cobas Influenza A/B (Roche) is cleared and CLIA-waived by FDA for use with nasopharyngeal swabs only. Xpert Xpress Flu is cleared and CLIA-waived by FDA for use with nasopharyngeal swabs and nasal swabs. Xpert Xpress Flu/RSV is cleared for use with nasopharyngeal swabs but is not CLIA-waived.

[f] Reverse transcription–polymerase chain reaction, including FDA-approved test systems, reference laboratory testing using analyte-specific *reagent* or laboratory-developed reagents. Some approved molecular assays can produce results in approximately 60 minutes to 80 minutes.

Adapted from Centers for Disease Control and Prevention. Influenza virus testing methods. 2018. Available at: https://www.cdc.gov/flu/professionals/diagnosis/table-testing-methods.htm. Accessed October 22, 2018.

nose or the back of a patient's throat and then sends the specimen for analysis. Result times vary on all of the testing methods.

Sometimes it is difficult for the HCP to collect an appropriate, uncontaminated influenza specimen. The CDC has a helpful visual guide for specimen collection that may be useful,[23] at https://www.cdc.gov/flu/pdf/professionals/flu-specimen-collection-poster.pdf.

Patient education is a patient's right and the HCP's responsibility.[24] For individuals diagnosed with SI, it is important to educate them about the potential complications that can arise and lead to hospitalization and even death.

Potential Complications

Recovery from mild SI generally is in a few days to less than 2 weeks unless symptoms are severe or complications develop. Depending on the age and usual health status of the individual, complications can be moderate to serious/severe (life threatening). Complications can result from the influenza virus itself or from invasive bacteria while compromised with influenza.

Moderate infections complications include[10]
- Bronchitis
- Ear
- Sinus

Serious/severe complications include
- Dehydration
- Inflammation
  - Encephalitis (brain)
  - Myocarditis (heart)
  - Myositis (muscle tissue)
  - Rhabdomyolysis (skeletal muscle)
- Multiple organ failure
  - Kidney
  - Respiratory
- Pneumonia
- Sepsis

Special Populations

Related to the normal immune system changes during pregnancy, pregnant women are more likely to develop serious influenza complications than healthy nonpregnant women. The risk continues up to 2 weeks postpartum.[25] The developing fetus is also susceptible to influenza complications in utero. Pertinent information is available for and about pregnant women at https://www.cdc.gov/flu/pdf/freeresources/pregnant/flushot_pregnant_factsheet.pdf.

Children less than 2 years of age are at a higher risk for developing influenza-related complications than children 5 years of age and older.[26] Resources for parents and caregivers of children are at https://www.cdc.gov/flu/parents/index.htm. Individuals under the age of 19 who have been on long-term aspirin therapy and people with a body mass index of 40 or more (morbid obesity) also are at risk for developing complications from influenza.[1]

From a cultural perspective, American Indians and Alaska Natives are at high risk for influenza complications.[27] The CDC has a comprehensive 2017 infographic available at https://www.cdc.gov/flu/resource-center/freeresources/graphics/aian.htm, specific to these 2 cultures. There are no evidence-based specific data on the why of this susceptibility other than social determinants of health linked to environment (born/live), economic (work), and social (play) factors that lead to reduced access to and use of health care services.[28]

Individuals with SI and preexisting conditions can have exacerbations of their disease states (see **Box 2**).

Individuals ages 65 years and older are at greater risk for influenza complications related to normal aging immune system changes. Chronic conditions also increase with age so these 2 factors double the risk of influenza complications. Older adults living in nursing homes and other long-term care (LTC) facilities also are at higher risk. Some researchers believe current vaccines are less effective in LTC residents with chronic comorbid conditions.[29] The American Nurses Association recommended flu vaccination of all health care personnel beginning in 2015.[30] In a September 6, 2018, press release, AMDA—The Society for Post-Acute and Long-Term Care Medicine recommended mandatory annual flu vaccines for all health care personnel who have direct or indirect contact with individuals in postacute care and LTC, unless contraindicated.[31] The Gerontological Society of America advocates making vaccinations a condition of hire in postacute care and LTC facilities.[32]

MANAGEMENT

Patients with mild SI symptoms should be educated on interventions/strategies they can use to weather uncomfortable SI symptoms (**Box 5**).

The World Health Organization analyzes yearly Northern Hemisphere influenza surveillance data and recommends the composition of the influenza vaccines for the following flu season. Because the World Health Organization does not have regulatory authority over vaccines in the United States, the Food and Drug Administration (FDA) convenes an annual meeting of the Vaccines and Related Biological Products Advisory Committee. This group reviews safety, immunogenicity, and effectiveness data

---

Box 5
Education for patients with mild influenza symptoms

- Cover mouth and nose with a tissue/handkerchief or arm/elbow when coughing or sneezing
  - Throw tissues in the trash immediately after using
  - Handkerchiefs should be replaced and laundered frequently
- Frequent handwashing
- If fever present—stay home for at least 24 hours after temperature returns to normal baseline (usual for the individual)
- Limit personal (face-to-face) contact with others
- Rest
- Keep warm
- Drink plenty of fluids—especially water
- Avoid alcohol
- Stop smoking
- Eat nutritious snacks and meals throughout the day
- If contracting SI and living alone—let a friend, family member, or neighbor know of illness
- Seek out health care if not getting better or if having a preexisting chronic condition (frailty in older adults, high temperature for 4–5 days, symptoms worsening, or developing shortness of breath or chest pain)[10]

and then finalizes the virus composition of the influenza vaccines manufactured in the United States for the next season.[4]

The priority evidence–based recommendation for the 2018 to 2019 influenza season is routine annual vaccination for individuals (without contraindications) beginning at 6 months of age or older. Factors to consider related to vaccination include the following[4,33]:

- Timing of the vaccination is important, related to the unpredictable start, peak, and decline of the virus season.
  - The optimal time to offer vaccinations is when they become available and prior to the onset of influenza activity in the community.
  - Vaccinations should be administered prior to the end of October.
    - Providing vaccinations later in the year can still be beneficial for minimizing symptoms.
    - For children ages 6 years to 8 years requiring 2 doses in a season, the vaccine should be administered as soon as it is available; the second dose is administered at 4 weeks or later.
  - Vaccinations can be administered throughout the flu season, but revaccination is not recommended.
  - HCPs should take every opportunity to offer and recommend the vaccine during annual examinations, acute visits, or even hospitalizations.
- High-risk (for potentially severe influenza complications) individuals should be vaccinated first.
- Individuals/caregivers/family members living with or providing care for persons at high-risk for complications should be vaccinated. This category includes (not all-inclusive).
  - Health care professionals/employees/staff working in primary care and acute care, LTC, assisted living, subacute rehabilitation, foster and group homes, childcare and adult day care programs, congregate meal centers, community health departments, emergency response teams, low-income housing, urgent care, and so forth.
  - Professional students, such as those in nursing, medicine, social work, therapy (physical, occupational, and speech), nutrition, and counseling
  - Clergy, religious leaders, and lay visitors
  - Household caregivers/workers/contacts, including babysitters, nannies, day care employees, and home care personnel
  - Volunteers in any type of facility/organization where they might come in contact with individuals at increased risk for influenza complications

Vaccinations

Over the years, research has led to the development and production of different types of vaccinations for different people and circumstances. Selection of the appropriate product is based on age, risk factors, and other special circumstances, such as egg allergy, pregnancy, history of Guillain-Barré syndrome after influenza, and immunocompromised persons.[4] It is imperative that HCPs know a person's unique story to make a correct decision about vaccine type.

For the current 2018-2019 flu season, a component of the B/Victoria was changed and the influenza A (H3N2) component was updated.[34] A quadrivalent (4-component) live, attenuated influenza vaccine (LAIV) was made available as a nasal spray this flu season as well.[34] The vaccine has been approved for nonpregnant individuals ages 2 years to 49 years.[34]

The information the CDC collects from studying genetic changes in influenza viruses plays an important public health role by helping to determine whether existing vaccines and antiviral drugs will work against new influenza viruses. The CDC also helps determine the potential for influenza viruses in animals to infect humans[7] (**Fig. 3**).[35] For a summary of the US vaccine recommendations of the Advisory Committee on Immunization Practices, see https://www.cdc.gov/flu/pdf/professionals/acip/acip-2018-19_summary-of-recommendations.pdf.[36]

Antiviral Medication

Prescription antiviral medications are second-line defense and work against SI viruses.[22,33] These medications are not a substitute for an influenza vaccine. The duration of symptoms is reduced by 1 day if an antiviral is started within 2 days of exhibiting SI symptoms; potential complications also may be reduced.[22] Even after 4 days to 5 days of SI symptom onset, severe symptoms can be reduced by starting an antiviral.[17] There are 3 FDA-approved antiviral drugs (neuraminidase inhibitors) recommended by the CDC to treat SI in the current 2018 to 2019 season[10,22]:

- Oseltamivir: available as a generic version or under the trade name Tamiflu—both are available as a pill or liquid suspension; causes gastrointestinal symptoms; should be taken with food; approved for early treatment in individuals 14 days

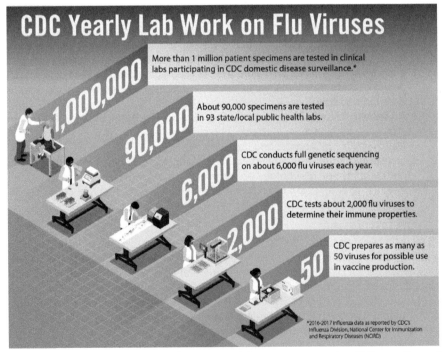

Fig. 3. Infographic demonstrating the rigorous laboratory process the CDC goes through every year in analyzing previous year's viral specimens to determine the components of the next flu season. (*Adapted from* Centers for Disease Control and Prevention. CDC yearly lab work on flu viruses infographic. 2017. Available at: https://www.cdc.gov/flu/resource-center/freeresources/graphics/infographic-lab-work.htm. Accessed October 21, 2018.)

and older; generally prescribed twice a day for 5 days; hospitalized patients or older adults in LTC may take for longer periods of time; cost is approximately $130 for a full course[36,37]

- Peramivir: trade name Rapivab; intravenously given by an HCP 1 time over 15 minutes to 30 minutes; early treatment of SI in people 2 years of age and older[36,37]
- Zanamivir: trade name Relenza; inhaled powder; approved for people 7 years of age and older; not recommended for individuals with asthma or chronic obstructive pulmonary disease; generally prescribed twice a day for 5 days; hospitalized patients or older adults in LTC may take for longer periods of time; cost is approximately $65 without insurance for a full course[36,37]

Common complications from these medications are nausea and vomiting.[22] In the current flu season, the circulating SI viruses are resistant to adamantane antiviral drugs (amantadine and rimantadine) and are not recommended for symptom management.[20]

Contraindications

Determining who should not receive an influenza vaccination requires knowing a person's story and social and medical histories as well as values and life goals. Individuals who should not be vaccinated include those with a history of severe reaction to a prior influenza vaccination, those who have a life-threatening allergy to the vaccine or any ingredient in the vaccine components, children less than 6 months of age, and individuals who are ill at the start of the vaccination season (although, when well, may receive the vaccine) (**Table 2**).

Antibiotics are for the treatment of bacteria that lead to infections; they are not appropriate in the treatment of viruses or SI. Prescribing an antibiotic for SI may lead to future resistance to harmful bacteria. Practicing diligent antibiotic stewardship is prudent and saves health care dollars. If the individual has an ear infection or sinus infection during SI, antibiotics are appropriate.

IMPLICATIONS FOR PRACTICE

It is the duty of all HCPs to advocate for the health and welfare of human beings across the life span, doing everything in their power to prevent illness, in particular, this killer virus. To maximize prevention and patient education, all HCPs should[32]

- Assess the immunization status of every patient during every practice encounter
- Share evidence-based recommendations for vaccines that every patient needs
- Debunk the many myths and misconceptions that exist related to vaccinations
- Administer required vaccines or refer to an HCP who can immunize
- Document all vaccines administered or received by patients
- Receive an annual influenza vaccination
- Encourage clinic staff and front-line workers to receive annual influenza vaccinations; consider making yearly flu vaccines mandatory for employment in the practice
- Respect SI as a potentially dangerous virus that can lead to increased mortality and morbidity

Together, HCPs can have a positive impact on the future of SI not only in the United States but also globally. Advocating for changes in health care policies related to cost of vaccinations and supporting immunization research can have a remarkable impact on improving quality of life for all peoples of the world.

Table 2
Contraindications and precautions to the use of influenza vaccines: United States, 2018–2019 influenza season[4,a]

Vaccine Type	Contraindications	Precautions
IIV	History of severe allergic reaction to any component of the vaccine[b] or after a previous dose of any influenza vaccine	Moderate or severe acute illness with or without fever History of Guillain-Barré syndrome within 6 wk of receipt of influenza vaccine
RIV	History of severe allergic reaction to any component of the vaccine	Moderate or severe acute illness with or without fever History of Guillain-Barré syndrome within 6 wk of receipt of influenza vaccine
LAIV	History of severe allergic reaction to any component of the vaccine[b] or after a previous dose of any influenza vaccine Concomitant aspirin-containing or salicylate-containing therapy in children and adolescents Children aged 2 y through 4 y who have received a diagnosis of asthma or whose parents or caregivers report that an HCP has told them during the preceding 12 mo that their child had wheezing or asthma or whose medical record indicates a wheezing episode has occurred during the preceding 12 mo Children and adults who are immunocompromised due to any cause (including immunosuppression caused by medications or by HIV infection) Close contacts and caregivers of severely immunosuppressed persons who require a protected environment Pregnancy Receipt of influenza antiviral medication within the previous 48 h	Moderate or severe acute illness with or without fever History of Guillain-Barré syndrome within 6 wk of receipt of influenza vaccine Asthma in individuals aged ≥5 y Other underlying medical conditions that might predispose to complications after wild-type influenza infection (eg, chronic pulmonary, cardiovascular [except isolated hypertension], renal, hepatic, neurologic, hematologic, or metabolic disorders [including diabetes mellitus])

Abbreviations: ACIP, Advisory Committee on Immunization Practices; IIV, inactivated influenza vaccine; RIV, recombinant influenza vaccine.

[a] Immunization providers should check FDA-approved prescribing information for 2018 to 19 influenza vaccines for the most complete and updated information, including (but not limited to) indications, contraindications, and precautions. Package inserts for US-licensed vaccines are available at https://www.fda.gov/BiologicsBloodVaccines/Vaccines/ApprovedProducts/ucm093833.htm.

[b] History of severe allergic reaction (eg, anaphylaxis) to egg is a labeled contraindication to the use of IIV and LAIV. ACIP recommends, however, that any licensed, recommended, and age-appropriate influenza vaccine (IIV, RIV, or LAIV) may be administered to persons with egg allergy of any severity (see Persons with a History of Egg Allergy for further recommendations and information).

Adapted from Grohskopf LA, Sokolow LZ, Broder KR, et al. Prevention and control of seasonal influenza with vaccines: recommendations of the advisory committee on immunization practice-United States, 2018-19 influenza season. MMWR Recomm Rep 2018;67(3):1–20. Available at: https://www.cdc.gov/mmwr/volumes/67/rr/rr6703a1.htm#T1_down.

REFERENCES

1. Centers for Disease Control and Prevention, National Center for Immunization and Respiratory Diseases. Seasonal influenza (flu). 2018. Available at: https://www.cdc.gov/flu/about/disease/high_risk.htm. Accessed October 20, 2018.
2. Centers for Disease Control and Prevention. Key facts about influenza (flu). 2018. Available at: https://www.cdc.gov/flu/keyfacts.htm. Accessed October 20, 2018.
3. World Health Organization. Influenza virus infections in humans. 2014. Available at: http://www.who.int/influenza/human_animal_interface/virology_laboratories_and_vaccines/influenza_virus_infections_humans_feb14.pdf. Accessed October 20, 2018.
4. Grohskopf LA, Sokolow LZ, Broder KR, et al. Prevention and control of seasonal influenza with vaccines: recommendations of the advisory committee on immunization practice-United States, 2018-19 influenza season. MMWR Recomm Rep 2018; 67(3):1–20. Available at: https://www.cdc.gov/mmwr/volumes/67/rr/rr6703a1.htm#T1_down. Accessed October 21, 2018.
5. Torrey T. The difference between an epidemic and a pandemic: how the definitions direct the public health response. 2018. Available at: https://www.verywellhealth.com/difference-between-epidemic-and-pandemic-2615168. Accessed October 20, 2018.
6. Epocrates. Seasonal influenza infection: epidemiology. 2018. Available at: https://online.epocrates.com/diseases/623/Seasonal-influenza-infection/Epidemiology. Accessed October 21, 2018.
7. Centers for Disease Control and Prevention. Influenza virus genome sequencing and genetic characterization. 2017. Available at: https://www.cdc.gov/flu/professionals/laboratory/genetic-characterization.htm. Accessed October 21, 2018.
8. Clancy S. Genetics of the influenza virus. Nature Ed 2008;1(1):83.
9. World Health Organization. A revision of the system of nomenclature for influenza viruses: a WHO memorandum. 1980. Available at: https://www.ncbi.nlm.nih.gov/pmc/articles/PMC2395936/pdf/bullwho00427-0070.pdf. Accessed October 20, 2018.
10. American Lung Association. Lung health & diseases. 2018. Available at: https://www.lung.org/lung-health-and-diseases/lung-disease-lookup/influenza/. Accessed October 21, 2018.
11. Centers for Disease Control and Prevention. Types of influenza viruses. 2017. Available at: https://www.cdc.gov/flu/about/viruses/types.htm. Accessed October 21, 2018.
12. Dolin R, Hirsch MS, Thorner AR. Epidemiology of influenza 2018. Available at: https://www.uptodate.com/contents/epidemiology-of-influenza. Accessed October 21, 2018.
13. Centers for Disease Control and Prevention. How the flu virus can change: drift and shift. 2017. Available at: https://www.cdc.gov/flu/about/viruses/change.htm. Accessed October 21, 2018.
14. Centers for Disease Control and Prevention. 2018-19 Advisory Committee on Immunization Practices (ACIP). Background. 2018. Available at: https://www.cdc.gov/flu/professionals/acip/2018-2019/background/background-epidemiology.htm. Accessed October 21, 2018.
15. World Health Organization. Risk factors. 2018. Available at: http://www.who.int/topics/risk_factors/en/. Accessed October 20, 2018.
16. Nordqvist C. All you need to know about flu. Medical News Today 2017. Available at: https://www.medicalnewstoday.com/articles/15107.php. Accessed October 21, 2018.

17. Agarwal D, Schmader KE, Kossenkov AV, et al. Immune response to influenza vaccination in the elderly is altered by chronic medication use. Immun Ageing 2018;15(19). https://doi.org/10.1186/s12979-018-0124-9.

18. Rote NS. Infection. In: McCance KL, Huether SE, editors. Pathophysiology: the biologic basis for disease in adults and children. 8th edition. St Louis (MO): Elsevier; 2019. p. 289–322.

19. Centers for Disease Control and Prevention. 10 things you need to know about childhood immunizations. 2018. Available at: https://www.cdc.gov/vaccines/vac-gen/10-shouldknow.htm. Accessed October 21, 2018.

20. World Health Organization. Influenza (seasonal): the pathogen. Available at: http://www.who.int/news-room/fact-sheets/detail/influenza-(seasonal). Accessed October 20, 2018.

21. Hart AM. Respecting influenza: an evidence-based overview for primary care nurse practitioners. J Nurse Pract 2015;1(1):41–8.

22. Centers for Disease Control and Prevention. What you should know about flu antiviral drugs. 2018. Available at: https://www.cdc.gov/flu/antivirals/whatyoushould.htm. Accessed October 19, 2018.

23. Centers for Disease Control and Prevention. Information for clinicians on influenza virus testing: information specimen collection visual guide. Available at: https://www.cdc.gov/flu/pdf/professionals/flu-specimen-collection-poster.pdf. Accessed October 21, 2018.

24. Dreeben O. Patient education in rehabilitation. Burlington (MA): Jones & Bartlett Learning; 2015.

25. Centers for Disease Control and Prevention. Pregnant women and influenza (flu). Available at: https://www.cdc.gov/flu/protect/vaccine/pregnant.htm. Accessed October 21, 2018.

26. Centers for Disease Control and Prevention. Children, the flu, and the flu vaccine. Available at: https://www.cdc.gov/flu/protect/children.htm. Accessed October 21, 2018.

27. Centers for Disease Control and Prevention. American Indians and Alaska Natives (AI/ANs) are at high risk for flu complications. Available at: https://www.cdc.gov/flu/resource-center/freeresources/graphics/aian.htm. Accessed October 21, 2018.

28. Indian Health Service, U.S. Department of Health and Human Services. American Indians, Alaska Natives and the flu. Available at: https://www.ihs.gov/forpatients/healthtopics/influenza/aianflu/. Accessed October 07, 2018.

29. Lansbury LE, Brown CS, Nguyen-Van-Tam JS. Influenza in long-term care facilities. Influenza Other Respir Viruses 2017;11:356–66.

30. Rittle C. What's new for influenza and zoster vaccines. Am Nurse Today 2018; 13(10). Available at: https://www.americannursetoday.com/influenza-zoster-vaccines/.

31. AMDA Releases Updated Recommendations on Annual Influenza Vaccination for Health Care Personnel. Available at: https://paltc.org/newsroom/amda-releases-updated-recommendations-annual-influenza-vaccination-health-care-personnel. Accessed October 21, 2018.

32. The Gerontological Society of America. Charting a path to increase immunization rates in the post-acute and long-term care settings. Available at: https://navp.org/images/navp/PDF/ImmunizRatesWP_FNL.pdf. Accessed October 21, 2018.

33. Lewnard JA, Cobey S. Immune history and influenza vaccine effectiveness. Vaccines (Basel) 2018;6(28) [pii:E28].

34. Centers for Disease Control and Prevention. Frequently asked flu questions 2018-2019 influenza season 2018. Available at: https://www.cdc.gov/flu/about/season/flu-season-2018-2019.htm. Accessed October 21, 2018.

35. Centers for Disease Control and Prevention. CDC yearly lab work on flu viruses infographic. 2017. Available at: https://www.cdc.gov/flu/resource-center/freeresources/graphics/infographic-lab-work.htm. Accessed October 21, 2018.

36. Prevention and control of seasonal influenza with vaccines: recommendations of the Advisory Committee on Immunization Practices (ACIP) – Unites States, 2018-19. Summary of recommendations. Available at: https://www.cdc.gov/flu/pdf/professionals/acip/acip-2018-19_summary-of-recommendations.pdf. Accessed October 21, 2018.

37. Bulloch M. Managing and preventing influenza with antivirals: information that may not be familiar. Pharm Times 2018. Available at: https://www.pharmacytimes.com/contributor/marilyn-bulloch-pharmd-bcps/2018/03/managing-and-preventing-influenza-with-antivirals-information-that-may-not-be-familiar-. Accessed October 21, 2018.

38. Leland DS, Ginocchio CC. Role of cell culture for virus detection in the age of technology. Clin Microbiol Rev 2007;20:49–78.

Recognition and Management of Malaria

Cynthia Gerstenlauer, ANP-BC, GCNS-BC, CDE, CCD

KEYWORDS

- Malaria • Mosquito transmitted • Vectors • Plasmodium • Chemoprophylaxis

KEY POINTS

- Malaria is one of the most severe public health problems in the world.
- Every traveler needs an individual assessment of their malaria risk.
- Travelers can protect themselves from malaria by taking prescription medicine, preventing mosquito bites, and through symptom awareness.
- Health care providers must be aware that malaria in febrile travelers is frequently misdiagnosed; health care providers must obtain a compete travel history on all patients with clinical infectious features.
- Malaria control efforts are limited by our incomplete understanding of *Plasmodium* and the complex relationships between human populations and the multiple species of mosquito and parasites.

INTRODUCTION

Malaria is one of the most severe public health problems in the world. It is a leading cause of death and disease in many developing countries. The most vulnerable are persons with little or no immunity against the disease, like young children, pregnant women, persons with asplenia, and travelers or migrants coming from areas with little or no malaria transmission.[1] Also at risk are long-term travelers who may elect to not take malaria chemoprophylaxis, or those visiting friends and relatives in their home country because they are less likely to seek pretravel advice.[2]

The costs of malaria to individuals, families, communities, and governments are enormous. Costs to individuals and their families include preventive measures, purchase of drugs, expenses for travel to and treatment at medical facilities, lost days of productivity, travel insurance, and expenses for burial in case of death. Costs to governments and communities include maintenance, supply, and staffing of health facilities; purchase of drugs and supplies; and public health interventions against

C. Gerstenlauer has no financial disclosures or any relationship with a related commercial company.
Troy Internal Medicine, 4600 Investment Drive, Troy, MI 48098, USA
E-mail address: cgerstenlauer@comcast.net

malaria, such as insecticide spraying or distribution of insecticide-treated bed nets. Direct costs like illness treatment, and premature death, have been estimated to be at least US$12 billion per year.[3] The cost in lost economic growth is many times more than that.

EPIDEMIOLOGY

According to the World Health Organization's World Malaria Report 2016 and the Global Malaria Action Plan, 3.2 billion people (one-half of the world's population) live in areas at risk of malaria transmission in 106 countries and territories.[1] In 2016, malaria caused an estimated 216 million clinical episodes, and 445,000 deaths; most were young children in sub-Saharan Africa.[1] An estimated 91% of deaths in 2016 were in the World Health Organization African Region.[1] The Centers for Disease Control and Prevention (CDC) helped to eliminate malaria as a major public health problem in the United States in the late 1940s.[1] Outbreaks of locally transmitted cases of malaria in the United States have been small and relatively isolated, but the potential risk for the disease to reemerge is present owing to the abundance of competent vectors, especially in the West and Southeastern States.[3] Every year, millions of US residents travel to countries where malaria is present. On average, 29 additional cases have been reported in the United States each year since 1973.[3] In 2013, more than 1700 cases of imported malaria, including 10 deaths, diagnosed in the United States and its territories were reported to the CDC.[3] Of these, 82% were acquired in Africa, 11% in Asia, 6% in the Caribbean and the Americas, and 1% in Oceania.

MALARIA TRANSMISSION

Malaria occurs mostly in poor, tropical and subtropical areas of the world (**Fig. 1**). The full text of the malaria assessment and prophylaxis recommendation for a country can be found under the CDC map by clicking on the individual country. These maps are

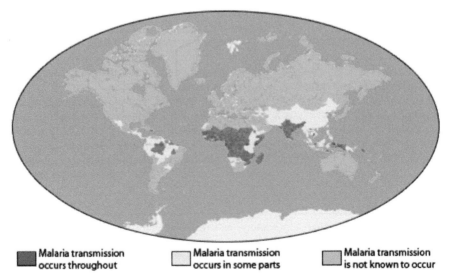

Malaria transmission occurs throughout

Malaria transmission occurs in some parts

Malaria transmission is not known to occur

Fig. 1. The CDC's map shows an approximation of the parts of the world where malarial transmission occurs. (*From* Centers for Disease Control and Prevention. Where Malaria Occurs. Available at: https://www.cdc.gov/malaria/about/distribution.html. Accessed March 14, 2019.)

meant to complement the Malaria Information and Prophylaxis by Country Table on the CDC's web site (https://www.cdc.gov/malaria/travelers/country_table) as well as the information currently available on the CDC Travelers' Health web site (https://wwwnc.cdc.gov/travel). Assessments of malaria endemicity are based largely on national surveillance reports and display assessments of the presence of malaria at the national and provincial level, not the city level. Malaria endemicity changes over time and so it is important to access the latest map.[3]

Africa is the most affected continent owing to a combination of factors[1]:

- A very efficient mosquito (*Anopheles gambiae*) is responsible for the high transmission rate.
- The predominant parasite species is *Plasmodium falciparum*, which is the species that is most likely to cause severe malaria and death.
- Local weather conditions often allow transmission to occur year round.
- Scarce resources and socioeconomic instability have hindered efficient malaria control activities.

Travelers to sub-Saharan Africa have the greatest risk of both getting malaria and dying from their infection.[1] However, all travelers to countries where malaria is present may be at risk for infection and death.

In other areas of the world, malaria is a less prominent cause of death, but can cause substantial disease and incapacitation, especially in rural areas of some countries in South America and South Asia. In areas with lower transmission (such as Latin America and Asia), residents are infected less frequently. Many persons may reach adult age without having built protective immunity and are thus susceptible to the disease, including severe and fatal illness.

MALARIA TRANSMISSION

Malaria in humans is caused by protozoan parasites of the *Plasmodium* genus: *Plasmodium falciparum, Plasmodium vivax, Plasmodium ovale,* or *Plasmodium malariae.*[3] *P ovale* has recently been shown by genetic methods to consist of 2 subspecies, *P ovale curtisi* and *P ovale wallikeri. Plasmodium knowlesi*, a zoonotic parasite of Eastern Hemisphere monkeys, has been documented as a cause of human infections and some deaths in Southeast Asia. *P falciparum* and *P vivax* are responsible for most malarial infections, and *P falciparum* causes the most severe form of malaria, along with the majority of deaths from malaria.

All species are typically transmitted by the bite of an infective female *Anopheles* mosquito. An *Anopheles* mosquito can only infect a person with malaria if it has already bitten a person with malaria. Less commonly, transmission can also occur by blood transfusion, organ transplantation, needle sharing, or congenitally from mother to fetus. Airport malaria refers to malaria caused by infected mosquitoes that are transported by aircraft from a malaria-endemic country to a nonendemic country. If the local conditions allow their survival, they can bite local residents who can thus acquire malaria without having traveled abroad. At the request of the states, the CDC assists in these investigations of locally transmitted mosquito-borne malaria. Malaria is a nationally notifiable disease.

LIFE CYCLE OF MALARIA

The life cycle of malaria parasites is complex and differs depending on the type of infection. [4] An understanding of the parasite's life cycle is necessary to understand both how the infection manifests and the way in which malaria prevention and treatment work at the different stages of the parasite's life cycle.

Fig. 2 shows the life cycle of the parasites of the *Plasmodium* genus that are causal agents of malaria. Malaria parasites infect 2 types of hosts: humans and female *Anopheles* mosquitos. Transmission begins with the development of sexual forms of the parasite, known as gametocytes, in an infected human host, and their

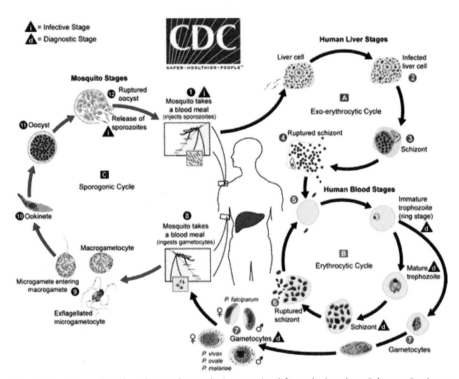

Fig. 2. The life cycle of malaria. The malaria parasite life cycle involves 2 hosts. During a blood meal, a malaria-infected female *Anopheles* mosquito inoculates sporozoites into the human host ❶. Sporozoites infect liver cells ❷ and mature into schizonts, which rupture and release merozoites ❸. (Of note, in *Plasmodium vivax* and *Plasmodium ovale* a dormant stage [hypnozoites] can persist in the liver and cause relapses by invading the bloodstream weeks, or even years later.) After this initial replication in the liver (exoerythrocytic schizogony Ⓐ), the parasites undergo asexual multiplication in the erythrocytes (erythrocytic schizogony Ⓑ). Merozoites infect red blood cells ❺. The ring stage trophozoites mature into schizonts, which rupture, releasing merozoites ❻. Some parasites differentiate into sexual erythrocytic stages (gametocytes) ❼. Blood stage parasites are responsible for the clinical manifestations of the disease. The gametocytes, male (microgametocytes) and female (macrogametocytes), are ingested by an *Anopheles* mosquito during a blood meal ❽. The parasites' multiplication in the mosquito is known as the sporogonic cycle Ⓒ. While in the mosquito's stomach, the microgametes penetrate the macrogametes generating zygotes ❾. The zygotes in turn become motile and elongated (ookinetes) ❿ that invade the midgut wall of the mosquito where they develop into oocysts ⓫. The oocysts grow, rupture, and release sporozoites ⓬, which make their way to the mosquito's salivary glands. Inoculation of the sporozoites ❶ into a new human host perpetuates the malaria life cycle. (*From* Centers for Disease Control and Prevention. Available at: https://www.cdc.gov/malaria/about/biology/index.html.)

subsequent transfer to an *Anopheles* mosquito after a blood meal. In humans, after the parasites enter the bloodstream, they travel to the liver and grow and multiply quickly. In most forms of malaria, some parasites stay in the liver to multiply and others flow into the red cells of the blood. Successive offsprings of parasites grown inside the red cells destroy them, releasing daughter parasites called merozoites, that continue the cycle by invading other cells. The blood stage parasites are those that cause the symptoms of malaria. The malaria parasites that stayed in the liver also continue to reproduce and send more parasites into the blood. After 10 to 18 days, the parasites are found (as sporozoites) in the mosquito's salivary glands. When the *Anopheles* mosquito takes a blood meal on another human, the sporozoites are injected with the mosquito's saliva and start another human infection when they parasitize the liver cells. Thus, the mosquito acts as a vector, carrying the disease from one human to another. The mosquito itself does not suffer from the presence of the parasites. This process of malaria results in repeated attacks of symptoms each time the malaria parasites are released into the blood. In humans, symptoms generally occur 12 to 20 days after the parasite has entered the blood. In the blood, the parasite's replication cycle lasts approximately 49 hours, causing a tertian fever that spikes approximately every 49 hours as newly replicated parasites erupt out of red blood cells.

CASE STUDY

A 47-year old man presents to the office with symptoms of fever, fatigue, chills, myalgias, and headaches for the past week. He denies experiencing nausea or vomiting, abdominal pain, jaundice, rhinorrhea, shortness of breath, or cough. He reports returning from Ghana on business 3 weeks ago and admits he did not take an antimalarial drug. He had sought travel health 3 months previously for travel to India and took atovaquone/proguanil, but owing to this being a short trip of 4 days, he did not think it was necessary. He had the recommended vaccines on board, including yellow fever and typhoid fever, because he had traveled to Kenya last year. His past medical history was unremarkable and noncontributory with no known drug allergies. His only medication included atorvastatin 20 mg/d.

Vital sign findings included a blood pressure of 140/72 mm Hg, pulse 88 beats/min, respiratory rate of 18/min, and a temperature of 100.4°F. Oxygen saturation with room air was 98%. His physical examination assessment findings were within normal limits.

The estimated relative risk of malaria for US travelers to Ghana is high. Malaria species includes *Plasmodium falciparum* 90%, *P ovale* 5% to 10%, and *P vivax* rare.[5] Chemoprophylaxis is recommended for all travelers, either mefloquine, atovaquone/proguanil, or doxycycline may be given.

Laboratory tests included a complete blood cell count, comprehensive metabolic panel, and blood smears to screen for malaria parasites. Thick and thin blood films were performed, processed immediately, and were read within a few hours. The result was positive for infection with *P ovale,* and the patient was determined to have uncomplicated malaria. His complete blood cell count and comprehensive metabolic panel were within normal limits. Infections with *P ovale* are generally sensitive to chloroquine. However, there is resistance to chloroquine in Ghana, and so the patient was treated with atovaquone/proguanil 250/100 mg 4 tablets by mouth daily for 3 days. The patient returned for a follow-up visit 72 hours later. Blood smears were repeated and were negative for the presence of malaria parasites. However, the patient was cautioned that with a history of *P ovale*, a dormant stage (hypnozoites) can persist in the liver and cause relapses by invading the bloodstream weeks or even years later.[3]

CLINICAL PRESENTATION AND DIAGNOSIS

Malaria must be recognized promptly to treat the patient in time and to prevent further spread of infection in the community via local mosquitoes. A delay in diagnosis and treatment is a leading cause of death in patients with malaria in the United States. Making a diagnosis of malaria begins with taking a thorough personal and family medical history, including symptoms and travel history, and completing a physical examination. Recent travel to subtropical or tropical areas of the world is an important clue that may increase the suspicion of a diagnosis of malaria.

Symptoms of malaria can develop as early as 8 to 10 days or up to a year or longer after a person has been bitten and infected with the parasite.[5] Most travelers who develop malaria are ill within a few weeks or up to 1 to 2 months after their return home. Some, however, do not become ill until 6 months or longer after their trip if they have been infected with forms of the parasite that persist in the liver, where commonly used prophylactic drugs may be ineffective.[5] Symptoms of malaria are characterized as a flulike illness with fever, chills, headache, myalgias, and, in some cases, abdominal pain and diarrhea, which initially may suggest other diagnoses.[5] A febrile illness with nonspecific symptoms could be influenza, malaria, dengue, typhoid fever, or rickettsial disease, among others. A diagnosis of malaria can easily be missed or delayed in areas of the world, such as the United States, where it is rare. Health care providers (HCPs) may not be familiar with the disease. Clinicians seeing a patient with malaria may forget to consider malaria among the potential diagnoses and not order the needed diagnostic tests. Malaria can result in anemia and jaundice. In severe disease, seizures, mental confusion, kidney failure, acute respiratory distress syndrome, coma, and death may occur. The remains of the destroyed red blood cells clump together and cause blockages in the blood vessels. This process can result in brain damage or kidney damage, which is potentially fatal.[3] Fever is the most frequently encountered symptom, and the presence of fever with or without other symptoms in a traveler returning from a malaria-endemic region requires that malaria be considered and excluded, even if the correct chemoprophylactic drugs have been properly taken.[5,6]

When evaluating a patient with a probable travel-related illness, the provider should consider the items summarized in **Box 1**.

Physical findings are typically nonspecific, depending on the degree of illness. Splenomegaly may be present. Note the level of alertness, any difficulty breathing, diaphoresis, and neurologic signs. Malaria can be suspected based on the patient's travel history, symptoms, and the physical findings on examination. However, a clinical diagnosis of malaria is unreliable, and clinicians are unable to distinguish malaria from other causes of fever.[6] For a definitive diagnosis to be made, laboratory tests must demonstrate the malaria parasites or their components.

Diagnostic testing includes taking a blood sample and examining a blood smear under a microscope. Before examination, the specimen is stained (most often with the Giemsa stain) to give the parasites a distinctive appearance. This technique remains the gold standard for laboratory confirmation of malaria.[3] However, it also depends on the quality of the reagents, of the microscope, and on the experience of the laboratorian. If the initial smear is negative for the plasmodia parasites but malaria is still suspected, blood smears should be repeated at least several times during the next day, especially if no other cause for the fever has been found.[3] A complete blood cell count can detect anemia. A comprehensive metabolic panel can detect hypoglycemia, renal failure, hyperbilirubinemia, and acid–base disturbances.

Box 1
Important medical history in an ill returned traveler

- Severity of illness
- Travel itinerary and duration of travel
- Timing of onset of illness in relation to international travel
- Past medical history and medications
- History of a pretravel consultation
  - Immunizations given
  - Adherence to malaria chemoprophylaxis
- Individual exposures
  - Type of accommodations
  - Mosquito precautions
  - Insect bites
  - Medical care while overseas (such as injections, transfusions)

Adapted from Fairley JK. Post-Travel Evaluation In: Brunette GW, editor. Centers for Disease Control and Prevention. CDC yellow book 2018: health information for international travel. New York: Oxford University Press; 2017. p. 496.

The CDC recommends that all cases of malaria diagnosed in the United States should be evaluated for evidence of drug resistance.[3] Drug resistance tests must be performed in specialized laboratories to assess the susceptibility to antimalarial compounds of parasites collected from a specific patient. Two main laboratory methods are available. The first is in vitro tests where the parasites are grown in culture in the presence of increasing concentrations of drugs. The drug concentration that inhibits parasite growth is used as the endpoint. The second is molecular characterization, where molecular markers assessed by polymerase chain reaction or gene sequencing also allow the prediction, to some degree, of resistance to some drugs.

Various test kits are available to detect antigens derived from malaria parasites. Such immunologic (immunochromatographic) tests most often use a dipstick or cassette format and provide results in 2 to 15 minutes. These rapid diagnostic tests (RDTs) offer a useful alternative to microscopy in situations where reliable microscopic diagnosis is not available. RDTs have been shown to decrease overdiagnosis and improve the targeting of antimalarials.[7] Malaria RDTs are currently used in some clinical settings and programs. This RDT is approved for use by hospital and commercial laboratories, not by individual clinicians or by patients themselves. It is recommended that all RDTs be followed up with microscopy to confirm the results and, if positive, to quantify the proportion of red blood cells that are infected. The use of this RDT may decrease the amount of time that it takes to determine that a patient is infected with malaria.

MALARIA PREVENTION

Malaria remains endemic in many countries, and travelers can protect themselves from malaria by taking prescription medicine and preventing mosquito bites (**Box 2**). Chemoprophylaxis is the best method of prevention. The drugs do not prevent the initial infection through a mosquito bite, but they do prevent the development of malaria parasites in the blood, which are the forms that cause disease. This type of prevention is also called suppression. All recommended chemoprophylaxis regimens involve taking a medication before, during, and after travel to an area with malaria. Starting the drug before travel allows the antimalarial agent to be in the blood before the traveler is exposed to malaria parasites.

Box 2
What can travelers do to prevent malaria?

Take prescription medication if recommended for your destination.
- Talk to your HCP about which medicine is best for you.
- Take this medicine before, during, and after your trip as directed.

Prevent mosquito bites.
- Cover exposed skin by wearing long-sleeved shirts, long pants, and hats.
- Use an appropriate insect repellent as directed. If you are also using sunscreen, apply sunscreen first and insect repellent second.
- Higher percentages of active ingredient provide longer protection. Use products with the following active ingredients.
  - DEET (N,N-Diethyl-meta-toluamide) 20% to 40%; products containing DEET include Off!, Cutter, Sawyer, and Ultrathon.
  - Picaridin (also known as KBR 3023, Bayrepel, and icaridin); products containing picaridin include Cutter Advanced, Skin So Soft Bug Guard Plus.
  - Oil of lemon eucalyptus or PMD (p-menthane-3,8-diol); products containing oil of lemon eucalyptus include Repel and Off! Botanicals.
  - IR3535; products containing IR3535 include Skin So Soft Bug Guard Plus Expedition and SkinSmart.
- Use permethrin-treated clothing and gear (such as boots, pants, socks, and tents). You can buy pretreated clothing and gear or treat them yourself.
  - Treated clothing remains protective after multiple washings. See the product information to find out how long the protection will last.
  - If treating items yourself, follow the product instructions carefully.
  - Do not use permethrin directly on skin.
- Avoid being outdoors from dusk to dawn.
- Stay and sleep in screened or air-conditioned rooms.
- Use an insecticide-treated bed net if the area where you are sleeping is exposed to the outdoors.

From Centers for Disease Control and Prevention. Malaria. Available at: https://wwwnc.cdc.gov/travel/diseases/malaria. Accessed March 14, 2019.

Chemoprophylaxis guidelines do not recommend one drug versus another, but individualize the treatment based on past experience, country of travel, itinerary, possible drug interaction, potential side effects, costs, and medical contraindications.[3] The drugs used for antimalarial chemoprophylaxis are generally well-tolerated. However, side effects can develop. Minor side effects usually do not require stopping the drugs. Travelers with serious side effects should talk to their HCP to determine if the symptoms are related to the medicine and make a medication change. Chemoprophylaxis can be started earlier if there are concerns about tolerating a medication.[3] If unacceptable side effects develop, there would be time to change the medication before the traveler's departure. The daily antimalarial drugs have short half-lives; if the traveler is late by 1 to 2 days, protective blood levels are less likely to be maintained.[3] The weekly drugs have longer half-lives, and so offer the advantage of a wider margin of error if the traveler is late with a dose.[3] **Table 1** lists the available drugs for chemoprophylaxis in the United States. The HCP need to be very familiar with these drugs to prescribe them appropriately. The contraindications and adverse effects listed are not exhaustive. Additional information about choosing a malaria chemoprophylaxis regime can be found at www.cdc.gov/malaria/traveler/drugs.html.

Chemoprophylaxis is recommended for all travelers visiting malarious areas. However, if travelers elect to not take chemoprophylaxis, or are unable to take, or develop symptoms consistent with malaria, travelers can use presumptive self-treatment

Table 1
Antimalarial drugs for chemoprophylaxis

Generic/Trade Name (Manufacturer)	Adult Dosing	Contraindications and Precautions	Adverse Effects
Atovaquone/proguanil (Malarone, GlaxoSmithKline)	1 tablet 250 mg/100 mg once daily, 1–2 d before arriving in the malarial area, daily while there, and 7 d after leaving the malarial area. Efficacy (>95% for *Plasmodium falciparum* and *vivax*)	Should not be used with severe renal impairment (clearance <30 mL/min) Dose of oral anticoagulant may need to be reduced or monitoring of PT may need to be more often Cannot be used by women who are pregnant or breastfeeding a child that weighs <5 kg.	Mild headache, GI complaints Take with food or whole milk. If vomits within 30 min of taking a dose, repeat the dose
Chloroquine phosphate (Aralen and generic, Abbott Laboratories)	1 tablet 500 mg once weekly, 1–2 wk before travel in the malarial endemic area, weekly throughout the stay, and 4 wk after travel	Cannot be used in areas with chloroquine or mefloquine resistance. Use limited by widespread *P falciparum resistance*: all malarious areas except Central America West of the Panama Canal Zone, Mexico, Haiti (some recent resistance reported), the Dominican Republic, and most the of the Middle East (some resistance reported in Yemen, Oman and Iran) Must use IM (not intradermal) route for rabies vaccination Interaction with other drugs like acetaminophen	Occasional GI disturbances, vomiting, headache, dizziness, blurred vision, insomnia and pruritis Exacerbation of psoriasis, eczema, and other exfoliative dermatoses

(continued on next page)

Table 1
(continued)

Generic/Trade Name (Manufacturer)	Adult Dosing	Contraindications and Precautions	Adverse Effects
Doxycycline (Vibramycin and generic)	1 tablet or capsule 100 mg once daily, 1–2 d before arriving in the malarial area, throughout the stay in endemic areas and 28 d after travel Efficacy (84%–98% for *P falciparum*)	Multiple interactions (alcohol, anticoagulants, sulfonylureas, phenytoin, carbamazepine, antacids, bismuth) Cannot take simultaneously with oral typhoid vaccine Contraindicated in children <8 y, pregnancy, allergy to tetracycline Do not take within 3 d of oral typhoid Do not take at bedtime (esophagitis, ulcers) Interaction with alcohol, anticoagulants, oral contraceptives, others	Photosensitivity (<10%), vaginal candidiasis GI complaints (dyspepsia, vomiting) reduced with taking with meals Hepatotoxicity
Mefloquine (Larium and generic, Roche)	1 tablet 250 mg once weekly, 1–2 wk before travel in the malarial endemic area, weekly while there, and 4 wk after returning home. Efficacy (>90%) against all *Plasmodia sp.)* Safety	Cannot be used in areas with mefloquine resistance (*P falciparum* resistance in Southeast Asia Some resistance in China, Amazon region, parts of sub-Saharan Africa, Haiti) Mefloquine should not be given to anyone with a history of seizures, psychiatric illness (active or recent depression, generalized anxiety disorder, psychosis, schizophrenia, other major psychiatric disorders), cardiac conduction disorders (Personal or family history of QT prolongation, bradycardia, ventricular arrhythmias), or allergy to mefloquine or related compounds (quinine or quinidine) Caution for severe renal or hepatic impairment Recent MI, CHF	Frequent: vertigo, lightheadedness, nausea, vomiting, other GI disturbances, nightmares, visual disturbances, sleep disturbances Occasional: confusion Rare: psychosis, hypotension, convulsions, coma, paresthesia's, hepatotoxicity, visual illusions, hallucinations, depression

| Primaquine generic | 30 mg orally, daily
Begin 1–2 d before travel to malarious areas
Take daily at the same time each day while in the malarious area and for 7 d after leaving such areas | Travel to areas with primarily *P vivax* | Contraindicated in people with severe G6PD deficiency, pregnancy and lactation, unless the infant being breastfed has a documented normal G6PD level
Myelosuppression, SLE, RA
Caution mild-mod G6PD deficiency, electrolyte abnormalities, personal or family history QT prolongation, ventricular arrhythmias, bradycardia, recent MI, CHF | Hemolytic anemia, leukopenia, QT prolongation, methemoglobinemia
Nausea, vomiting, epigastric discomfort, abdominal cramps, dizziness, rash, pruritus |

Abbreviations: CHF, congestive heart failure; GI, gastrointestinal; IM, intramuscular; MI, myocardial infarction; PT, prothrombin time; RA, rheumatoid arthritis; SLE, systemic lupus erythematosus.

From Centers for Disease Control and Prevention. Choosing a Drug to Prevent Malaria. Available at: https://www.cdc.gov/malaria/travelers/drugs.html. Accessed March 14, 2019.

(**Table 2**). The CDC recommends atovaquone/proguanil for presumptive self-treatment, but it cannot be used if the traveler took this drug as chemoprophylaxis. If atovaquone/proguanil cannot be used because of contraindications or other

Table 2			
Drug for presumptive self-treatment of malaria			
Generic/Trade Name (Manufacturer)	**Adult Dosing**	**Contraindications and Precautions**	**Adverse Effects**
Atovaquone/ proguanil Malarone (GlaxoSmithKline) 250 mg/100 mg	4 tablets once daily (can be divided into 2 doses) for 3 d Efficacy >95% for *Plasmodium falciparum* and *vivax* and for multidrug-resistant *P falciparum*	Not for those taking Malarone prophylaxis If cannot be used, the CDC Malaria Hotline (770-488-7788) can provide support	As in **Table 1**
Artemether-lumefantrine Coartem (Novartis) 20 mg/120 ng	A total of 6 tablets over 3 d; initial dose, second dose 8 h later, then 1 dose twice daily for 2 d	Treatment of uncomplicated *Plasmodium falciparum* malaria infections; not for treatment of severe malaria or prevention Not for people on mefloquine prophylaxis Not recommended for pregnant women, and women breastfeeding infants weighing <5 Personal or family history QT prolongation Ventricular arrhythmias, bradycardia, recent MI, CHF Severe renal or hepatic impairment	Bullous dermatitis, QT prolongation Headache, anorexia, dizziness, asthenia, arthralgia, myalgia, nausea, fever, rigors, sleep disorders, palpitations, vomiting, abdominal pain, fatigue, hepatomegaly, splenomegaly, diarrhea, cough, insomnia, anemia, malaise, pruritus, rash, vertigo, aspartate aminotransferase elevated
Primaquine	30 mg orally daily for 14 d if borderline G6PD deficient, give 45 mg orally daily	As in **Table 1**	
			(continued on next page)

Table 2 (continued)			
Generic/Trade Name (Manufacturer)	**Adult Dosing**	**Contraindications and Precautions**	**Adverse Effects**
Quine sulfate plus doxycycline	Quine sulfate 650 mg every 8 h for 3–7 d plus doxycycline 100 mg twice daily for 7 d	Quinine: black box warning hematologic toxicity Hypersensitivity to mefloquine, quinidine, pregnancy, breastfeeding, G6PD deficiency, myasthenia gravis. QT prolongation, recent MI, CHF, etc	Give with food Serious: cinchonism, QT prolongation, arrhythmias, angioedema, bronchospasm, other serious reactions Headache, vasodilation, diaphoresis, nausea, tinnitus, impaired hearing, dizziness, blurred vision, altered color perception, fever/rigors, other GI, photosensitivity

Abbreviations: CHF, congestive heart failure; GI, gastrointestinal; MI, myocardial infarction.

Adapted from Centers for Disease Control and Prevention. Guidelines for Treatment of Malaria in the United States. Based on drugs currently available for use in the United States – updated July 1, 2013. Available at: https://www.cdc.gov/malaria/diagnosis_treatment/treatment.html.

considerations, consult a travel medicine expert or call the CDC Malaria Hotline for other potential options for self-treatment.

Long-term travelers who may not have access to medical care should bring along medications for emergency self-treatment should they develop symptoms suggestive of malaria, such as fever, chills, headaches, and muscle aches, and cannot obtain medical care within 24 hours.

Per US Food and Drug Administration recommendations, travelers to malaria-endemic areas should be informed that they may not donate blood for 1 year after travel.[3] Former residents of malaria-endemic areas may not donate blood for 3 years after departing or within 3 years if revisiting. Persons diagnosed with malaria may not donate blood for 3 years after treatment.

MALARIA TREATMENT

If a traveler has symptoms of malaria while abroad, it is best to seek medical attention while there, and not get on the next commercial flight back to the States for treatment. The disease can progress rapidly, and medical treatment would not be available in transit (eg, at 30,000 feet). Travelers should be informed that malaria could be fatal if treatment is delayed. All forms of malaria can be associated with significant illness, and *Plasmodium falciparum* can be fatal if diagnosis and appropriate treatment are not prompt.[5] Suspected or confirmed malaria, especially *P falciparum*, is a medical emergency, requiring urgent intervention because clinical deterioration can occur rapidly and unpredictably. Travelers should also be informed that malaria could be fatal even when treated, which is why it is always preferable to prevent malaria cases rather than rely on treating infections after they occur.

It is possible to obtain adequate treatment for malaria even in a country with a poor health care infrastructure. However, locating a reputable HCP can be more complicated, and cultural and language barriers can compound the situation. Travelers should be counseled on how they can find reputable medical facilities at their destination, such as using the International Society of Travel Medicine web site (www.istm.org), the American Society of Tropical Medicine and Hygiene web site (www.astmh.org), or the International Association for Medical Assistance to Travelers (www.iamat.org). The traveler can also contact the US embassy or consulate in their host country to ask for a clinician recommendation or call a family member in the United States themselves and ask the family to do this for them. A US consular officer can assist in locating medical services and informing family or friends (see www.Travel.State.Gov). In some countries, the traveler may need to travel to the capital or a major city to access better care. Medical evacuation is another option, but can be pricey; evacuation insurance needs to be purchased in advance.

The treatment of malaria depends on many factors, including disease severity, the species of malaria parasite causing the infection, and the part of the world in which the infection was acquired. The latter 2 characteristics help to determine the probability that the organism is resistant to certain antimalarial drugs. Additional factors such as age, weight, and pregnancy status may limit the available options for malaria treatment.

If a patient has an illness suggestive of severe malaria and a compatible travel history in an area where malaria transmission occurs, it is advisable to start treatment as soon as possible, even before the diagnosis is established.[2] Antimalarial drugs are also used in the treatment of malaria. CDC recommendations for malaria treatment can be found at www.cdc.gov/malaria/diagnosis_treatment/index.html.

EFFORTS TO ERADICATE MALARIA

Within the last decade, increasing numbers of partners and resources have rapidly increased malaria control efforts. This scale-up of interventions has saved 3.3 million lives globally and decreased malaria mortality by 45%, leading to hopes and plans for elimination and ultimately eradication.[1] The CDC brings its technical expertise to support these efforts with its collaborative work in many malaria-endemic countries and regions.

To continue to prevent illness and deaths owing to malaria, the CDC works within this country by:

- Administering the national Malaria Surveillance System
- Investigating instances of locally transmitted malaria (eg, transfusion malaria)
- Preventing malaria among international travelers
- Consulting with clinicians and providing advice on the diagnosis and treatment of malaria in the United States
- Providing artesunate for the treatment of severe cases of malaria in the United States
- Advising blood collection centers

Today's malaria control efforts are limited by our incomplete understanding of the biology of *Plasmodium* and of the complex relationships between human populations and the multiple species of mosquito and parasites. A Consultant Panel on Basic Science and Enabling Technologies was convened in 2009 to help accelerate progress toward malaria disease elimination and ultimately, eradication.[8] The project is called the Malaria Eradication Research Agenda. The recommendations came from an extensive search of published and unpublished literature, and the expertise of the panel. Areas looked at included the *Plasmodium* life cycle in both the human host and the *Anopheles* vector, and included critical, unanswered questions about parasite transmission, human infection in the liver, asexual-stage biology, and malaria persistence. The panel believed an integrated approach encompassing human immunology, parasitology, and entomology, and using new and emerging biomedical technologies, offered the best approach to develop effective vaccines, drugs, and diagnostic tools. Since the first agenda for malaria eradication was published in 2011 and again in 2017, there has been progress toward this end, but more critical questions need to be answered with more research to be done and technologies developed.

MALARIA HOTLINE

The CDC is available on a 24-hour/365-day basis for HCP needing guidance on diagnosis and management of suspected cases of malaria.[3] Assistance can be provided through the CDC Malaria Hotline (770-488-7788) from 9:00 AM to 5:00 PM EST. The emergency after-hours hotline is 770-488-7100 and ask to page the person on call for the Malaria Branch. Guidance for the diagnosis and treatment of malaria is also available at the CDC's Malaria Diagnosis & Treatment web site (https://www.cdc.gov/malaria/). Using email to ask for clinical advice is not recommended, because it is not constantly monitored and there may be delays in answering.

SUMMARY

Despite the apparent progress in decreasing the global prevalence of malaria, many areas remain malaria endemic, and the use of prevention measures by travelers is still inadequate. *Anopheles* mosquitoes capable of transmitting malaria exist in the United States. Thus, there is a constant risk that malaria transmission can resume in the United States. Malaria is almost always preventable; failing to take malaria chemoprophylaxis and take mosquito prevention measures is linked to most cases of the disease. HCPs must be aware that malaria in febrile returned travelers is frequently misdiagnosed. For this reason, it is important for HCP to obtain a complete travel history on all returned travelers with clinical infectious features and with a history of travel or migration from malaria-endemic areas. Considering the diagnosis of malaria in febrile travelers with risk factors increases the likelihood of prompt diagnosis and treatment. Additionally, HCP need to know that the CDC can assist them in the diagnosis and management of patients with malaria. Travelers and HCP must be educated about the importance of malaria diagnosis, treatment, and prevention.

REFERENCES

1. Centers for Disease Control and Prevention. Malaria's Impact Worldwide. Available at: https://www.cdc.gov/malaria/malaria_worldwide/impact.html. Accessed September 11, 2018.
2. Shellvarajah M, Hatz C, Schlagenhauf P. Malaria prevention recommendations for risk groups visiting sub-Saharan Africa: a survey of European expert opinion and international recommendations. Travel Med Infect Dis 2017;19:49–55.
3. Arguin P, Tan K. Malaria. In: Brown CM, editor. CDC health information for international travel ("The yellow book"). 2018.
4. Centers for Disease Control and Prevention. Biology. Available at: https://www.cdc.gov/malaria/about/biology/index.html. Accessed October 14, 2018.
5. Centers for Disease Control and Prevention. Where Malaria Occurs. Available at: https://www.cdc.gov/malaria/about/distribution.html. Accessed March 14, 2019.

6. Lillie P, Duncan C, Sheehy S, et al. Distinguishing malaria and influenza: early clinical features in controlled human experimental infection studies. Travel Med Infect Dis 2012;10:192–6.

7. Leslie T, Mikhail A, Mayan I, et al. Rapid diagnostic tests to improve treatment of malaria and other febrile illnesses: patient randomized effectiveness trial in primary care clinics in Afghanistan. BMJ 2014;348:g3730.

8. Old 6 The malERA Refresh Consultative Panel on Basic Science and Enabling Technologies. malERA: an updated research agenda for basic science and enabling technologies in malaria elimination and eradication. PLoS Med 2017; 14(11):e1002451.

Lyme Disease

Amber Carriveau, DNP, FNP-BC*, Hanna Poole, BSN, RN,
Anne Thomas, PhD, ANP-BC, GNP

KEYWORDS

- Lyme disease • *B burgdorferi* • Deer tick • Erythema migrans • Tick-borne disease

KEY POINTS

- Timeliness of tick removal reduces likelihood of infection.
- Early recognition of erythema migrans with subsequent antibiotic treatment reduces chronic disease phase.
- Use of protective clothing, insect repellants, and avoidance of endemic tick-infested areas reduce incidence of Lyme disease.

INTRODUCTION

Lyme disease is the most commonly reported vector-borne disease in the United States and has been a nationally notifiable condition since 1991, with disease cases reported to local and state health departments by both clinicians and laboratories.[1] Lyme disease is found most frequently in the upper Midwest, Northeast, and mid-Atlantic regions[1] (**Fig. 1**); however, current surveillance data indicate that the geographic distribution of the disease is expanding into neighboring regions.[1] From 2008 to 2015, there were 208,834 confirmed and 66,755 probable cases reported to the Centers for Disease Control and Prevention (CDC), with the total number of confirmed cases remaining at more than 30,000 annually.[1] On average, 8344 annual probable cases were reported from 2008 to 2015, representing 48 states.[1] For all years, July is the peak month of illness-onset for confirmed and probable cases. The early summer months are when the nymphal stage of the vector ticks are seeking blood meal hosts.[1]

Information from surveillance data regarding the sex of confirmed and probable cases indicated that most cases were male individuals (56.7%). Information on race was available in only 62.1% of cases; of those, the vast majority were white (89.7%) followed by other race (6.8%), black (1.6%), Asian/Pacific Islander (1.5%), and American Indian/Alaska Native (<1%).[1] Patient age was available in 89.6% of the records

Disclosure Statement: The authors have no commercial or financial conflicts of interest and have no funding sources to disclose.
Michigan State University College of Nursing, Life Science Building, 1355 Bogue Street, #A228, East Lansing, MI 48824, USA
* Corresponding author.
E-mail address: carrive6@msu.edu

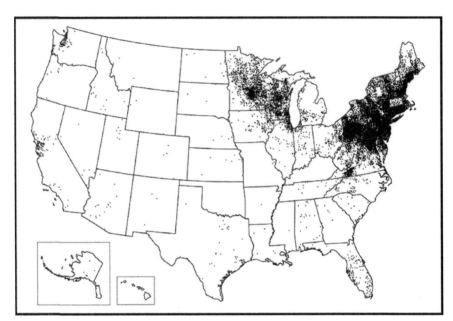

Fig. 1. Reported cases of Lyme disease. One dot placed randomly within county of residence for each confirmed case. (*From* CDC, Lyme disease: data and surveillance. Available at: https://www.cdc.gov/lyme/datasurveillance/maps-recent.html. Accessed February 6, 2019.)

and indicated a bimodal distribution with peaks at ages 5 to 9 years and 50 to 55 years.[1]

CAUSES

Lyme disease is commonly caused by the spirochete *Borrelia burgdorferi* in the United States.[2] This bacterial spirochete occurs most frequently in small vertebrates and is transmitted to humans via bites by the *Ixodes scapularis* or *Ixodes pacificus* ticks, commonly known as deer ticks or black-legged ticks.[3] Different strains of *Borrelia* have been identified through antibody testing, which has led to differences in clinical manifestations of the disease in the United States as compared with other parts of the world, particularly Europe.[3]

Disease transmission to humans requires the need for the tick to ingest a blood meal to transform to their next stage of development.[4] Ticks locate themselves in low-lying vegetation awaiting the host. Once attached to the host, the tick inserts its central piercing agent, called a hypostome, into the host's skin. *Ixodes* ticks secrete a cementing material to the skin for additional attachment, as well as anticoagulants, immunosuppressive, and anti-inflammatory substances. These substances allow the pathogens to pass to the host and also may alter the host's awareness to the tick bite.[4] Most tick bites do not result in the transmission of infection, and only 2% to 3% of all persons bitten by *Ixodes scapularis* ticks in endemic areas develop Lyme disease.[4] The tick needs to remain in place between 24 and 48 hours for transmission of the pathogen to occur.[5,6]

BORRELIA BURGDORFERI LIFE CYCLE

The infectious disease cycle of the bacterial spirochete known to cause Lyme disease involves colonization, infection of the genus *Ixodes* tick, then transmission to the host.

Although the *Ixodes* tick progresses through a 2-year life cycle encompassing 4 developmental stages, egg, larva, nymph, and adult, only the egg stage does not require a blood meal, and only ticks in the nymphal and adult stage transmit *B burgdorferi*. Ticks acquire the spirochete from feeding on an infected animal during the larvae, nymph, and adult stages. Interestingly, mice and deer are incompetent hosts for *B burgdorferi*, although they can carry the spirochete; thereby making the animals infested but not infected.[3]

The cycle begins with the adult tick laying its eggs each spring, which emerge as larvae in the summer. The larvae feed once, usually in the later summer on small invertebrates, such as mice or squirrels.[3,7] The nymph emerges from the larvae in the following spring and feeds on small invertebrates. The nymph molts into an adult tick the following fall, completing the 2-year life cycle, and feeds on larger animals, with deer being the preferred host.[3]

As noted previously, the risk of Lyme disease is highest in the late spring and early summer months when the nymphal-stage ticks are seeking their blood meal. Nymphs are responsible for 90% of the human disease transmission because of their abundance and the increase in human activity during that time.[3] In addition, the relatively smaller size of the nymph in comparison with the adult tick makes them harder to detect and remove before the time of transmission of 24 to 48 hours.[3,4]

CLINICAL PRESENTATION

Lyme disease presents in 1 of 3 general stages. Each stage has distinct symptomatology, although clinical features may overlap, contributing to difficulty in diagnosis.[8] The stages of Lyme disease are as follows: early localized disease, early-disseminated disease, and late-disseminated disease. The most common presentation is early localized disease.[9]

Early Localized Disease

In early localized disease, symptom onset develops anywhere from 3 to 30 days,[10] averaging 1 to 2 weeks, after a bite from an infected tick.[11–13] Erythema migrans (EM) is the classic sign of early infection, indicating a focal cutaneous infection.[6] The rash develops at the site of the tick bite and occurs in approximately 70% to 80% of patients.[13–15] Erythema migrans has a multitude of presentations, which contributes to the difficulty in establishing an accurate diagnosis. The EM rash, originally thought to be pathognomonic for Lyme disease, also has been found in patients with southern tick-associated rash illness, the etiology of which is yet unclear.[16] The classic "bull's eye" or targetlike presentation is present in only approximately 30% to 40% of cases.[13] An EM diagnosis requires that lesions be at least 5 cm in size.[17] The EM rash most commonly appears in the following areas: abdomen, axilla, inguinal area, and popliteal fossa.[13] However, in children, in addition to the previously noted locations, approximately one-quarter of tick bites are on the head and neck[18]; thus, care should be taken to examine the scalp and head, as hair could easily disguise the EM rash.[19]

EM may appear similar to a sunburn and may contain vesicular or necrotic areas.[11,13] The affected area may burn, itch, or be hot to the touch. The presence of surrounding lymphedema is also possible.[13] Other associated symptoms include flulike illness presenting as fever, headache, fatigue, myalgias, arthralgias, and anorexia.[8,14] Laboratory findings during this time may include leukocytosis, leukopenia, elevated erythrocyte sedimentation rate, thrombocytopenia, and liver function abnormalities.[14]

The differential diagnosis of EM includes cellulitis, varicella zoster, and herpes simplex.[20] It is not uncommon, particularly in pediatric patients, to develop a hypersensitivity reaction after a tick bite, which can be mistaken for EM.[14] The rash of EM gradually increases in size in the 24 to 48 hours following its appearance, whereas a hypersensitivity reaction will resolve within a few days and requires no treatment.[14] A close follow-up should be arranged for those presenting with an early rash smaller than 5 cm following a potential or known tick bite.[14]

Early-Disseminated Disease

Early-disseminated Lyme disease results from the untreated hematogenous spread of bacteria,[21] and typically occurs weeks to months after a bite from an infected tick.[10] Symptoms may include multiple EM lesions, or neurologic or cardiac symptoms. Neurologic symptoms occur in approximately 12.5% of adult and pediatric patients and include facial palsy, radiculoneuropathy, and rarely lymphocytic meningitis.[1] Facial palsy is the most common neurologic presentation, and involvement of the seventh cranial nerve is usually seen, although other cranial nerves may be involved.[1,9]

In pediatric patients, multiple EM lesions account for the most common presentation of early-disseminated disease.[19] The cranial nerve palsy that affects pediatric patients is similar to that of adults.[22] Meningitis and encephalitis rarely occur in both adults and children.[1,18] Lyme carditis is uncommon in both children and adults. According to the most recent surveillance data from the CDC, approximately 1.5% of patients had carditis on presentation.[1] These data were not separated by pediatric and adult patients, but prior studies have suggested that only 0.5% of children present with carditis.[18]

Late-Disseminated Disease

Late-disseminated disease develops months to years after an infected tick bite.[10] The most common presenting symptom in late-disseminated disease is Lyme arthritis, which accounted for almost 30% of presenting cases reported to the CDC.[1] Typical features of Lyme arthritis include a monoarthritis or oligoarthritis, characteristically affecting the knees, although other joints, both large and small, may be affected. Although Lyme arthritis shares a similar clinical presentation with other reactive arthritis syndromes and septic arthritis, some distinguishing features are present.[23] Fever is usually absent, large knee effusions are not uncommon, and, when present, typically do not cause the patient much discomfort, unlike the effusion seen in septic arthritis[23] (Table 1).

LABORATORY DIAGNOSTICS

Diagnostic testing for Lyme disease has proven challenging for several reasons. First, the B burgdorferi spirochete is only found in low numbers in infected tissue or fluids.[25] This has prompted the development of diagnostic testing aimed at detecting antibodies to the spirochete.[21]

The current recommendations for 2-step testing were the result of a working conference on the diagnostics of Lyme disease.[26] These guidelines are still in use and were recommended by the Infectious Diseases Society of America (IDSA) and supported by the CDC.[6,27] The first step is testing with an approved enzyme immunoassay (EIA) or immunofluorescence assay (IFA). Although both are approved first-step tests, the EIA has a greater ease of use, and thus is the more commonly ordered test.[27] The EIA measures the immunoglobulin (Ig)M and IgG antibody response to B burgdorferi antigens[26] and has high sensitivity. However, the EIA can cross-react with many other

Table 1
Summary of disease presentation

Stage	Clinical Presentation in Adults and Children	Diagnostic Testing
Early localized disease	EM, flulike symptoms.	No diagnostic testing is warranted in those presenting with classic EM rash
Early-disseminated disease	Carditis Neurologic disease • Cranial neuropathy • Most commonly seventh cranial nerve, • Peripheral neuropathy Multiple EM lesions Musculoskeletal symptoms	Two-step testing • EIA or IFA • If either are equivocal or positive, proceed to Western immunoblot
Late-disseminated disease	Arthritis	Two-step testing • EIA or IFA • If either are equivocal or positive, proceed to Western immunoblot
Post-Lyme disease syndrome (PLDS)	Myalgias, arthralgias, headache, neck pain, backache, fatigue, cognitive dysfunction, irritability	Rule out other potentially causative conditions; no diagnostic testing specific of Lyme disease should be performed unless acute infection is suspected

Abbreviations: EIA, enzyme immunoassay; EM, erythema migrans; IFA, immunofluorescence assay.
Data from Refs.[1,6,8,19,24,26]

antigens, decreasing its use as a stand-alone test and contributing to the difficulty in the development of accurate diagnostic testing.[25]

If the resulting EIA or IFA test is equivocal or positive, further testing with a Western immunoblot should be performed.[26] False positives with the EIA are not uncommon. The addition of the Western immunoblot decreases the likelihood of false-positive results and increases the specificity of the EIA to greater than 98%.[28] The Western immunoblot also detects antibodies to *B burgdorferi*; however, the antibodies tested are a specific set of protein antigens.[26] Similar to the EIA, cross-reactivity with other non-*Borrelia* antigens is not uncommon.[21] It is therefore imperative that the Western immunoblot results be interpreted according to the precise recommendations provided to ensure the most accurate interpretation is given. Overinterpretation of the antibody bands is a known source of potential misdiagnosis and decreased specificity of results.[29] Several other diagnostic tests are available and include polymerase chain reaction (PCR) and culture; however, they are rarely recommended in the clinical setting.[21]

Presentation with the classic EM rash is the only clinical situation in which the IDSA recommends treatment for Lyme disease without serologic testing.[6] Two-step serologic testing is not adequately sensitive during the first 2 weeks of infection to be diagnostically useful, thus is not recommended; however, this 2-week window is often the timeframe in which patients initially present with an EM rash.[25]

There are laboratory facilities that purport to offer more "accurate" interpretations of the Western blot. Interpretations of testing outside the recommendations by the IDSA have been found to significantly increase the potential for false-positive results, and the potential for harm that ensues from the resultant overdiagnosis.[6,30] Furthermore, testing for Lyme disease by culture or PCR of blood, cerebrospinal fluid, or tissue has been unreliable at best, and, with few exceptions, is not recommended in routine practice.[25]

Care should be taken to test only those patients with high clinical suspicion or increased risk. Given the limitations of the current testing algorithm, testing those at low risk or those with vague constitutional symptoms, such as malaise or fatigue, is likely to result in false-positive results and increase the likelihood of unwarranted antibiotic therapy, and the potential for subsequent antibiotic-induced side effects, with a very low likelihood of symptom improvement.[21]

LYME DISEASE TREATMENT
Early Localized Disease Treatment

Doxycycline is the gold standard treatment for adults in the early localized and early-disseminated phases of Lyme disease.[6] Clinicians should be aware that intermittent shortages of doxycycline may cause costs to be prohibitive for patients. In these cases, minocycline is proposed as an alternative.[31] Alternative therapies for tetracycline-allergic adults are available (**Table 2**).[12]

When starting antibiotic therapy, it is important to note that a Jarisch-Herxheimer (JH)-type reaction may occur in 7% to 30% of patients.[13,32,33] The JH-type reaction is characterized by sudden worsening of symptoms within 24 to 48 hours of antibiotic therapy initiation, and it is more likely to occur in individuals with multiple EM lesions.[13] Most affected individuals experience chills, an increased fever response, and a worsening rash, which typically resolves in a matter of hours.[13,33] However, some case reports include more dangerous sequelae, including hypotension, acute respiratory distress syndrome, uterine contractions in pregnancy, liver and kidney impairment, myocardial injury, meningitis, altered level of consciousness, seizure, and stroke.[32]

The mechanism for the JH-type response is not entirely understood. Researchers propose it is the result of a short-lived and rarely fatal inflammatory response involving cytokines, nonendotoxin pyrogens, and lipoproteins associated with the spirochete. In most patients, supportive care and hydration are sufficient until the JH-type response has resolved.[32]

Early-Disseminated Treatment

Lyme carditis treatment typically requires 14 to 21 days of oral doxycycline.[13] However, symptomatic heart blocks may be treated with intravenous (IV) antibiotics and monitoring in the hospital. In severe cases, temporary pacemakers are used to provide rhythm control.[6]

For managing Lyme meningitis, 14 days of oral doxycycline treatment demonstrates equivalent effectiveness and safety compared with IV ceftriaxone treatment. A similar approach is recommended for Lyme radiculopathy and cranial neuropathy. Corticosteroids can be used in addition to antibiotics to reduce neurologic manifestations of early-disseminated Lyme.[33] Other indications and treatments for early-disseminated Lyme disease are presented in **Table 2**.

Late-Disseminated Management

Lyme arthritis requires 28 days of either doxycycline, amoxicillin, or cefuroxime axetil. The 28-day cycle can be repeated once if pain is resistant to the first round of oral antibiotics. Alternatively, IV ceftriaxone may be attempted, but there is little evidence for the superiority of a second round of oral versus IV medications. Further rounds of antibiotics are not recommended for management of arthritis after the second

Table 2
Treatment for Lyme disease in adults

Indication	Drug	Dose	Route	Frequency	Duration
Early localized or early-disseminated disease with mild carditis[a,b]	Doxycycline OR	100 mg	PO	Twice daily	10–14 d (14–21 d if carditis present)
	Amoxicillin OR	500 mg	PO	Three times daily	14–21 d
	Cefuroxime axetil	500 mg	PO	Twice daily	14–21 d
Early-disseminated disease with neurologic symptoms (facial nerve palsy, radiculoneuropathy, or meningitis)	Doxycycline[c]	100 mg	PO	Twice daily	14–28 d
Early-disseminated disease with encephalitis or more severe carditis[d]	Ceftriaxone OR	2 g	IV	Daily	14–28 d
	Cefotaxime	2 g	IV	Every 8 h	14–28 d
Late-disseminated disease with arthritis and absence of neurologic symptoms	Doxycycline OR	100 mg	PO	Twice daily	28 d
	Amoxicillin	500 mg	PO	Three times daily	28 d
Persistent arthritis with minimal or no response to adequate oral therapy	Ceftriaxone OR	2 g	IV	Daily	14–28 d
	Doxycycline OR	100 mg	PO	Twice daily	28 d
	Amoxicillin	500 mg	PO	Three times daily	28 d

Abbreviations: IV, intravenous; PO, by mouth.

[a] Mild carditis is defined as first-degree atrioventricular (AV) block with PR interval less than 300 ms.

[b] Alternative, although less-effective therapies include the following: azithromycin 500 mg daily for 7 to 10 days, clarithromycin 500 mg twice daily for 14 to 21 days, and erythromycin 500 mg 4 times daily for 14 to 21 days.

[c] Alternative therapies include amoxicillin or cefuroxime for isolated facial nerve palsy. If doxycycline is contraindicated, therapy with IV ceftriaxone should be considered for other forms of early-disseminated disease.

[d] More severe carditis as defined as first-degree AV block with PR interval greater than or equal to 300 ms, second- or third-degree AV block, symptomatic patients: chest pain, dyspnea, or syncope.

Data from Wormser GP, Dattwyler RJ, Shapiro ED, et al. The clinical assessment, treatment, and prevention of Lyme disease, human Granulocytic anaplasmosis, and babesiosis: clinical practice guidelines by the Infectious Disease Society of America. Clin Infect Dis 2006;43:1089–134. Available at: https://doi.org/10.1086/508667. Accessed September 1, 2018; and Sanchez E, Vannier E, Wormser GP, et al. Diagnosis, treatment, and prevention of Lyme disease, human granulocytic anaplasmosis, and babesiosis. JAMA 2016;315:1767–77. Available at: https://doi.org/10.1001/jama.2016.2884. Accessed September 22, 2018.

attempt, but extended use of anti-inflammatory drugs and disease-modifying antirheumatic drugs are recommended with appropriate monitoring.[13,23,33] In some patients with persistent synovitis identified on MRI, a synovectomy may be helpful.[23]

Adverse drug reactions and antibiotic resistance have been observed with antibiotic treatments for Lyme disease extending past 28 days, with no additional benefits observed. Therefore, chronic, routine prescription of antibiotics is not recommended. Health care providers should consider specialist referrals appropriate for the patient's symptom profile.[2,11,12,33,34] Cognitive symptoms, fatigue, pain, and depression can be very disabling and distressing to patients, so a comprehensive approach to supportive care is critical.[35] Antidepressants, anti-inflammatory agents, a healthy diet, rest, and counseling have demonstrated some effectiveness in managing the effects of late-disseminated Lyme disease. More research is needed to support these interventions.[11]

Childhood Lyme Disease Treatment

Historically, treatment with doxycycline has been avoided in children younger than 8. Recently, the American Academy of Pediatrics has endorsed its use in this population, as long as treatment duration is ≤24 days.[36] Early-disseminated and late-disseminated presentations require longer treatment durations (**Table 3**).

EDUCATION AND PREVENTION
Prophylactic Antibiotics

Recent evidence indicates that a single 200-mg dose of doxycycline has been effective in preventing Lyme disease following a known *Ixodes* tick bite in adults. In the pediatric patient 8 years or older, a single 4-mg/kg dose of doxycycline is recommended, up to 200 mg. It should be noted that only recently the American Academy of Pediatrics has endorsed the use of doxycycline in children younger than 8.[36] Recommendations for oral prophylaxis have yet to be tested on children, and have been extrapolated to include children older than 8.[6] At this time, prophylactic treatment for children younger than 8 is not recommended.[6] Oral prophylaxis is advised only as long as the bite occurred in a tick-endemic area, the engorged tick is thought to have been attached for 36 hours, and the prophylactic antibiotic can be initiated within 72 hours of discovery of the tick.[11,13,34] As of the 2017 case definition, the CDC considers a high-incidence state to be one that has demonstrated 10 confirmed cases per 100,000 residents over the previous 3 reporting years.[37] See **Fig. 1** for the distribution of Lyme disease in the United States as of 2016.

Nausea is the most commonly reported adverse effect with the prophylactic approach, which currently demonstrates an efficacy of 87%.[11,13,34] To counter the possible adverse effects of prophylactic therapy, patients should be educated on the risks and signs of a *Clostridium difficile* infection and the preventative benefits of probiotic use. Patient preference should be taken into consideration and the risks and benefits of single-dose prophylactic treatment versus potential for development of infection should be discussed.[38,39]

Tick Avoidance

Health care providers should assess the types of activities in which patients participate, whether for work or leisure, in an effort to reduce exposure to ticks. Education should include times of peak tick activity, between May and October.[11,40] During these times, if possible, patients should avoid grassy and wooded endemic areas, as these are natural habitats for tick vectors of Lyme disease. It is also important for health care providers in nonendemic areas to screen for travel to endemic areas, and tailor education and monitoring activities accordingly.[6,19,41,42]

If patients wish to spend time outdoors in endemic areas, they should be encouraged to cover exposed skin and remain in the center of groomed trails if possible. Clothing can be treated with DEET or permethrin, according to package directions, before entering wooded and grassy areas. The use of DEET with children and pregnant or lactating women has been controversial, due to reports of seizures in children proximal to DEET application. However, Koren and colleagues[43] note that

Table 3
Treatment for Lyme disease in children

Indication	Drug	Dose	Route	Frequency	Duration	Maximum Dose
Early localized or early-disseminated disease with mild carditis[a,b]	Doxycycline OR	4.4 mg/kg per d	PO	Divided twice daily	10–21 d (14–21 d if carditis present)	100 mg per dose
	Amoxicillin OR	50 mg/kg per d	PO	Divided 3 times daily	14–21 d	500 mg per dose
	Cefuroxime axetil	30 mg/kg per d	PO	Divided twice daily	14–21 d	500 mg per dose
Early-disseminated disease with neurologic symptoms (facial nerve palsy, radiculoneuropathy, or meningitis)	Doxycycline	4.4 mg/kg per d	PO	Divided twice daily	14–28[d] d	100 mg per dose
Early-disseminated disease with severe neurologic symptoms; eg, encephalitis, or more severe carditis[c]	Ceftriaxone OR	50–75 mg/kg per d	IV	Once daily	14–28 d	2 g per dose
	Cefotaxime	150–200 mg/kg per d	IV	Divided 3 times daily	14–28 d	6 g per d
Late-disseminated disease with arthritis and absence of neurologic symptoms	Doxycycline OR	4.4 mg/kg per d: children ≥8 y of age	PO	Divided twice daily	28 d[d]	100 mg per dose
	Amoxicillin	50 mg/kg per d	PO	Divided 3 times daily	28 d	500 mg per dose
Persistent arthritis with minimal or no response to adequate oral therapy	Ceftriaxone OR	50–75 mg/kg per d	IV	Once daily	14–28 d	2 g per dose
	Doxycycline OR	4.4 mg/kg per d: children ≥8 y of age	PO	Divided twice daily	28 d[d]	100 mg per dose
	Amoxicillin	50 mg/kg per d	PO	Divided 3 times daily	28 d	500 mg per dose

Abbreviations: IV, intravenous; PO, by mouth.

[a] Mild carditis is defined as first-degree atrioventricular (AV) block with PR interval less than 300 ms.

[b] Alternative, although less-effective therapies include the following: azithromycin 10 mg/kg once daily for 7 to 10 d, clarithromycin 15 mg/kg per day divided into twice-daily dosage for 14 to 21 days, or erythromycin 50 mg/kg per day divided into 4 doses per day, for 14 to 21 days.

[c] More severe carditis defined as first-degree AV block with PR interval greater than 300 ms, second-degree or third-degree AV block, symptomatic patients: chest pain, dyspnea, or syncope.

[d] Historically the use of doxycycline has not been recommended in children younger than 8 years. The use of doxycycline in this population, for therapy duration of up to 21 days, has recently been endorsed by the American Academy of Pediatrics.

Data from Wormser GP, Dattwyler RJ, Shapiro ED, et al. The clinical assessment, treatment, and prevention of Lyme disease, human Granulocytic anaplasmosis, and babesiosis: clinical practice guidelines by the Infectious Disease Society of America. Clin Infect Dis 2006;43:1089–134. Available at: https://doi.org/10.1086/508667. Accessed September 1, 2018; and American Academy of Pediatrics. Lyme disease. In: Kimberlin DW, Brady MT, Jackson MA, et al, editors. Redbook: 2018 report of the committee on infectious diseases. 31st edition. American Academy of Pediatrics; 2018. p. 515.

the evidence does not support an increased risk in children. Likewise, the CDC and Environmental Protection Agency suggest that most repellents containing DEET are safe for individuals older than 2 months. They recommend that DEET be applied to children under the supervision of an adult, and that the eyes and mouth be avoided. No further protections concerning DEET are recommended concerning children, or pregnant or lactating women. However, DEET concentrations greater than 50% tend to plateau in efficacy, offering no greater increase in protected time.[43,44]

Patients should be encouraged to bathe or shower within 2 hours of spending time outside, and to dry exposed clothing on the hot setting in the dryer. If clothes are wet, they should be dried on hot for 1 hour. If clothes are dry, 10 minutes is all that is, needed to kill possible ticks,[11,13]

Tick Removal

Appropriate and prompt tick removal is a very effective measure for preventing transmission of tick-borne illness. Ticks must attach to a host for at least 36 hours for spirochete transmission to occur.[2,13,41] However, Kahl and colleagues[45] found in animal studies that Lyme disease could be transmitted from a tick attached for as few as 16 hours.[43]

Consequently, health care providers should recommend thorough skin checks after spending time outdoors in endemic areas during peak tick activity. Ticks are likely to attach in hard-to-see areas, such as the scalp, groin, and axilla.[2,13,41] Therefore, a partner should assist with skin inspections when possible. Nymphal ticks are the most likely to bite and transmit Lyme disease, and these are approximately the size of a poppy seed. It can be very difficult to detect these ticks.[34] See **Fig. 2** for a visual comparison of tick sizes.

Effective tick removal can be accomplished with fine-tip forceps, by grabbing the insect as close to the surface of the skin as possible and pulling straight up.[6,13] If forceps are not available, Snydman[13] recommends the use of a cloth or paper to protect the fingers.

Emerging Evidence

Chemical methods for tick removal have been proposed, including the application of gasoline, petroleum jelly, clear fingernail polish, and methylated spirits to the attached tick. Commercial tick-removal devices have also been developed, and were tested in

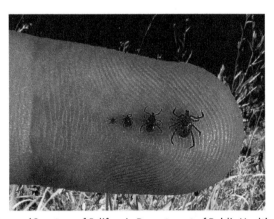

Fig. 2. Ticks on finger. (*Courtesy of* California Department of Public Health, Sacramento, CA.)

both human and animal studies. After a systematic review of tick-removal strategies, Guygelen and colleagues[46] concluded that the evidence for use of the commercial tick-removal devices and chemical tick removal is limited and currently of low quality. Therefore, tick removal using fine-tip forceps remains the standard of care until further studies are conducted.

DIAGNOSTIC AND TREATMENT CONTROVERSIES

Lyme disease diagnosis has been fraught with controversy and confusion since its identification by Dr Allen Steere in 1977.[47] Further research has since identified the causative spirochete and curative antibiotic therapy, although this has not quelled the debate. One of the more contentious areas of dispute surrounds the terms chronic Lyme disease versus post-Lyme disease syndrome (PLDS).

A small subset of patients that continued having vague symptoms that could not be explained by other medical conditions after appropriate treatment for serologic-positive Lyme disease was identified in the medical community. In response to this, the IDSA developed a definition for this clinical syndrome known as PLDS.[6] The definition was not meant to be a clinical diagnosis per se, but a more concrete description to aid in further study of this population.[35] Symptoms of PLDS include myalgias, arthralgias, head, neck and backache, fatigue, cognitive dysfunction, and irritibility.[48] The exact etiology of this constellation of symptoms is yet unclear. It is suggested to be the sequelae of a more severe case of Lyme disease, as those who are more ill on initial diagnosis have been found to be more likely to develop this syndrome.[49] PLDS also may be the result of the inflammatory response to the initial infection.[35] Regardless of the precise etiology, the IDSA is clear that PLDS does not constitute continued active infection, thus does not require retreatment or prolonged antibiotic therapy.[6]

In contrast, the International Lyme and Associated Diseases Society (ILADS) purports that PLDS does not accurately describe this syndrome and instead refers to this collection of symptoms as chronic Lyme disease. The exact definition of chronic Lyme disease by the ILADS is evasive at best, and it noted to be "an ongoing infection with any of the pathogenic bacteria in the *Borrelia burgdorferi sensu lato* group."[50] Using the ILADS definition, chronic Lyme disease could refer to patients with PLDS, those with serologic-positive active Lyme disease who did not complete a full course of appropriate antibiotic therapy, and patients lacking a serologic diagnosis of Lyme disease, with no history of tick bite or EM rash, and constitutional symptoms, such as fatigue and malaise, who have been given the diagnosis of chronic Lyme disease.

Several studies have been performed in an attempt to identify whether further treatment with IV, oral, or combination therapy was beneficial in this population, with mixed results. Although one study showed improvement in fatigue,[51] others did not.[52,53] In all studies using long-term antibiotic therapy, it is evident that this therapy contains risks. Several patients experienced side effects ranging from nuisance to life threatening.[51–53] Although no fatalities occurred in the previously noted studies, one cannot discount the deaths and near deaths that have been documented in patients being treated with long-term parenteral antibiotic therapy.[54,55]

It is evident that further study into PLDS is needed to determine what, if any, treatment will benefit patients with this diagnosis. Continued study into the expression of the *Borrelia* spirochete is also necessary to improve the limited diagnostics currently available. In the meantime, long-term antibiotic therapy should be reserved for patients with failure of active Lyme disease symptoms to remit with appropriate therapy and those with continued symptoms of active infection who have had an incomplete course of therapy on a case-by-case basis.[6]

SUMMARY

The incidence and geographic distribution of Lyme disease in the United States is steadily increasing. Patient education efforts that include information regarding protective clothing, tick removal, recognition of early signs and symptoms, and prompt treatment are a critical step in reducing the incidence of the disease. No vaccine for Lyme disease is currently available, which makes patient education paramount. Although effective treatments exist, Lyme disease can develop into a chronic disease with lifelong debilitating outcomes. Treatment controversy surrounds long-term antibiotic therapy for chronic Lyme disease. It is imperative that health care providers are knowledgeable about current treatment standards and recognize when referral to specialists is necessary.

REFERENCES

1. Schwartz AM, Hinckley AF, Mead PS, et al. Surveillance for Lyme disease – United States, 2008-2015. MMWR Surveill Summ 2017;66(SS-22):1–12. Available at: https://doi.org/10.15585/mmwr.ss6622a1. Accessed September 9, 2018.
2. Moore KS. Lyme disease: diagnosis, treatment guidelines, and controversy. J Nurse Pract 2015;11:64–9. Available at: https://doi.org/https://doi.org/10.1016/j.nurpra.2014.09.021. Accessed September 2, 2018.
3. Meyerhoff J, Diamond H, editors. Lyme disease. 2018. Available at: Emedicine.medscape.com. Accessed September 8, 2018.
4. Sanson T, Taylor J, editors. Tick-borne diseases. 2016. Available at: Emedicine.medscape.com. Accessed October 1, 2018.
5. Hu LT. In the clinic: Lyme disease. Ann Intern Med 2012;157(3):ITC2-2-2-16.
6. Wormser GP, Dattwyler RJ, Shapiro ED, et al. The clinical assessment, treatment, and prevention of Lyme disease, human Granulocytic anaplasmosis, and babesiosis: Clinical practice guidelines by the Infectious Disease Society of America. Clin Infect Dis 2006;43:1089–134. Available at: https://doi.org/10.1086/508667. Accessed September 1, 2018.
7. Ziegler R, Didas C, Smith J. Diagnosing and managing Lyme disease. JAAPA 2013;26(11):21–6.
8. Steere AC. Medical progress: Lyme disease. N Engl J Med 1989;321:586–96. Available at: https://www.nejm.org. Accessed September 22, 2018.
9. Steere AC. Lyme disease. N Engl J Med 2001;345:115–25. Available at: https://doi.org/10.1056/NEJM200107123450207. Accessed September 1, 2018.
10. Centers for Disease Control and Prevention. Signs and symptoms of untreated Lyme disease. 2016. Available at: https://www.cdc.gov/lyme/signs_symptoms/index.html. Accessed September 26, 2018.
11. Chaaya G, Jaller-Car JJ, Ali SK. Beyond the bull's eye: recognizing Lyme disease. J Fam Pract 2016;66:373–9. Available at: https://www.ncbi.nlm.nih.gov/pubmed/. Accessed October 1, 2018.
12. Sanchez E, Vannier E, Wormser GP, et al. Diagnosis, treatment, and prevention of Lyme disease, human granulocytic anaplasmosis, and babesiosis. JAMA 2016;315:1767–77. Available at: https://doi.org/10.1001/jama.2016.2884. Accessed September 22, 2018.
13. Snydman DR. Lyme disease. Medicine 2017;45:743–6. Available at: https://www.journals.elsevier.com/medicine. Accessed September 22, 2018.

14. Nadelman RB, Wormser GP. Lyme borreliosis. Lancet 1998;352:557–65. Available at: https://www.thelancet.com/journals/lancet/issues. Accessed September 9, 2018.

15. Steere AC, Sikand VK. The presenting manifestations of Lyme disease and the outcomes of treatment. N Engl J Med 2003;348:2472–3. Available at: https://www.nejm.org. Accessed September 1, 2018.

16. Masters EJ, Grigery CN, Masters RW. STARI, or Masters disease: LoneStar tick-vectored Lyme-like illness. Infect Dis Clin North Am 2008;22:361–76. Available at: https://doi.org/doi:10.1016/j.idc.2007.12.010. Accessed September 3, 2018.

17. Centers for Disease Control and prevention. Lyme disease – United States, 2003-2005. MMWR Morb Mortal Wkly Rep 2007;56(23):573–6. Available at: https://www.cdc.gov/mmwr/preview/mmwrhtml/mm5623a1.htm. Accessed October 15, 2018.

18. Gerber MA, Shapiro ED, Burge GS, et al. Lyme disease in children in southeastern Connecticut. N Engl J Med 1996;335:1270–4. Available at: https://www.nejm.org. Accessed September 26, 2018.

19. Sood SK. Lyme disease in children. Infect Dis Clin North Am 2015;29:281–94. Available at: https://doi.org/https://doi.org/10.1016/j.idc.2015.02.011. Accessed September 8, 2018.

20. Nadelman RB. Erythema migrans. Infect Dis Clin North Am 2015;29:211–39. Available at: https://doi.org/10.1016/j.idc/2015.02.001. Accessed September 9, 2018.

21. Moore A, Nelson C, Molins C. Current guidelines, common clinical pitfalls, and future directions for laboratory diagnosis of Lyme disease, United States. Emerg Infect Dis 2016;22:1169–77.

22. Belman AL, Iyer M, Coyle PK, et al. Neurologic manifestations in children with North American Lyme disease. Neurology 1993;43:2609–14. Available at: http://www.neurology.org. Accessed September 20, 2018.

23. Arvikar SL, Steere AC. Diagnosis and treatment of Lyme arthritis. Infect Dis Clin North Am 2015;29:269–80. Available at: https://doi.org/10.1016/j.idc.2015.02.004. Accessed September 12, 2018.

24. Nadelman RB, Nowakowski J, Forseter G, et al. The clinical spectrum of early Lyme borreliosis in patients with culture-confirmed erythema migrans. Am J Med 1996;100:502–8.

25. Aguero-Rosenfeld ME, Wang G, Schwartz I, et al. Diagnosis of Lyme borreliosis. Clin Microbiol Rev 2005;18:484–509. Available at: https://doi.or/10.1128/CMR.18.3.484?509.2005. Accessed August 28, 2018.

26. Centers for Disease Control and Prevention. Notice to readers: Recommendations for test performance and interpretation from the Second National Conference on Serologic Diagnosis of Lyme disease. MMWR Morb Mortal Wkly Rep 1995;44:590–7. Available at: https://www.cdc.gov/mmwr/preview/mmwrhtml/00038469.htm. Accessed October 10, 2018.

27. Centers for Disease Control and Prevention. Two-step laboratory testing process. 2015. Available at: https://www.cdc.gov/lyme/diagnosistesting/labtest/twostep/index.htm. Accessed September 9, 2018.

28. Craven RB, Quan TJ, Bailey RE, et al. Improved serodiagnostic testing for Lyme disease: results of a multicenter serologic evaluation. Emerg Infect Dis 1996;2:136–40. Available at: https://wwwnc.cdc.gov/eid/article/2/2/96-0211_article. Accessed August 28, 2018.

29. Centers for Diseases Control and Prevention. Notice to readers: caution regarding testing for Lyme disease. MMWR Morb Mortal Wkly Rep 2005;54:125. Available at: https://www.cdc.gov/mmwr/preview/mmwrhtml/mm5405a6.htm. Accessed September 22, 2018.

30. Aguero-Rosenfeld ME, Wormser G. Lyme disease: diagnostic issues and controversies. Expert Rev Mol Diagn 2015;15:1–4. Available at: https://doi.org/ http://www.tandfonline.com/action/showCitFormats?doi=10.1586/14737159. 2015.989837. Accessed August 29, 2018.
31. Carris NW, Pardo J, Montero J, et al. Minocycline as a substitute for doxycycline in targeted scenarios: a systematic review. Open Forum Infect Dis 2015;2(4). Available at: https://doi.org/10.1093. Accessed September 3, 2018.
32. Butler T. The Jarisch-Herxheimer reaction after antibiotic treatment of spirochetal infections: a review of recent cases and our understanding of pathogenesis. Am J Trop Med Hyg 2017;96(1):46–52.
33. Wormser GP, McKenna D, Nowakowski J. Management approaches for suspected and established Lyme disease used at the Lyme disease diagnostic center. Wien Klin Wochenschr 2016;130(15–16):463–7.
34. Patton SK, Phillips B. Lyme disease: diagnosis, treatment, and prevention: evidence-based strategies for nurses. Am J Nurs 2018;118(4):38–46. Available at: https://journals.lww.com/ajnonline/pages/default.aspx. Accessed September 14, 2018.
35. Lantos PM. Chronic Lyme disease. Infect Dis Clin North Am 2015;29:325–40. Available at: https://www.id.theclinics.com. Accessed September 20, 2018.
36. American Academy of Pediatrics. Lyme disease. In: Kimberlin DW, Brady MT, Jackson MA, et al, editors. Redbook: 2018 report of the committee on infectious diseases. 31st edition. Itasca (IL): American Academy of Pediatrics; 2018. p. 515.
37. Centers for Disease Control and Prevention. Lyme disease (*Borrelia burgdorferi*) 2017 case definition. Date unknown. Available at: https://wwwn.cdc.gov/nndss/ conditions/lyme-disease/case-definition/2017/. Accessed October 6, 2018.
38. Cameron DJ, Johnson LB, Maloney EL. Evidence assessments and guideline recommendations in Lyme disease: the clinical management of known tick bites, erythema migrans rashes and persistent disease. Expert Rev Anti Infect Ther 2014;12(9):1103–35.
39. Goldenberg JZ, Mertz D, Johnston BC. Probiotics to prevent *Clostridium difficile* infection in patients receiving antibiotics. JAMA 2018;320(5):499–500.
40. Lipsett S, Nigrovic LE. Diagnosis of Lyme disease in the pediatric acute care setting. Curr Opin Pediatr 2016;28:287–93. Available at: https://doi.org/https:// doi.org/10.1097/MOP.0000000000000339. Accessed August 30, 2018.
41. Borchers AT, Keen CL, Huntley AC, et al. Lyme disease: a rigorous review of diagnostic criteria and treatment. J Autoimmun 2015;57:82–115.
42. Novak C, Harrison A, Aucott J. Early disseminated Lyme disease with carditis complicated by post-treatment Lyme disease syndrome. Case Rep Infect Dis 2017;2017. Available at: https://doi.org/10.1155/2017/5847156. Accessed October 3, 2018.
43. Koren G, Matsui D, Bailey B. DEET-based insect repellents: safety implications for children and pregnant and lactating women. CMAJ 2003;169(3):209–12. Available at: www.cmaj.ca. Accessed September 29, 2018.
44. Mutebi J, Hawley WA, Brogdon WG. Protection against mosquitoes, ticks, & other arthropods. Available at: https://wwwnc.cdc.gov/travel/yellowbook/2018/the-pre-travel-consultation/protection-against-mosquitoes-ticks-other-arthropods. Accessed October 1, 2018.
45. Kahl O, Janetzki-Mittman C, Gray JS, et al. Risk of infection with *Borrelia burgdorferi* sensu lato for a host in relation to the duration of nymphal *Ixodes ricinus* feeding and the method of tick removal. Zentralbl Bakteriol 1998;287:41–52.

Available at: https://doi.org/10.1016/S0934-8840(98)80142-4. Accessed October 1, 2018.

46. Guygelen V, Borra V, DeBuck E, et al. Effective methods for tick removal: a systematic review. J Evid Based Med 2017;10:177–88.

47. Steere AC, Malawista SE, Snydman DR, et al. Lyme arthritis: an epidemic of oligoarticular arthritis in children and adults in three Connecticut communities. Arthritis Rheum 1977;20:7–17.

48. Logigian EL, Kaplan RF, Steere AC. Chronic neurologic manifestations of Lyme disease. N Engl J Med 1990;323:1438–44. Available at: https://doi.org/DO:10.1056/NEJM199011223232102. Accessed September 9, 2018.

49. Shadick NA, Phillips CB, Logigian EL, et al. The long-term clinical outcomes of Lyme disease: a population based retrospective cohort study. Ann Intern Med 1994;121:560–7. Available at: https://doi.org/10.7326/0003-4819-121-8-199410150-00002. Accessed September 7, 2018.

50. International Lyme and Associated Diseases Society. Controversies and challenges in treating Lyme and other tick-borne diseases. Date unknown. Available at: https://www.ilads.org/research-literature/controversies-challenges/. Accessed August 29, 2018.

51. Krupp LB, Hyman LB, Grimson R, et al. Study and treatment of post Lyme disease (STOP-LD): a randomized double masked clinical trial. Neurology 2003;60:1923–30. Available at: http://www.neurology.org. Accessed September 20, 2018.

52. Fallon BA, Keilp JG, Corbera KM, et al. A randomized, placebo-controlled trial of repeated IV antibiotic therapy for Lyme encephalopathy. Neurology 2008;70:992–1003. Available at: www.neurology.org. Accessed September 20, 2018.

53. Klempner MS, Hu LT, Evans J. Two controlled trials of antibiotic treatment in patients with persistent symptoms and a history of Lyme disease. N Engl J Med 2001;345:85–92. Available at: https://doi.org/10.1056/NEJM200107123450202. Accessed October 1, 2018.

54. Marks CM, Nawn JE, Caplow JA. Antibiotic treatment for chronic Lyme disease – Say no to the DRESS. JAMA Intern Med 2016;176(176):1745–6. Available at: https://doi.org/10.1001/jamainternmed.2016.6229. Accessed October 1, 2018.

55. Marzec NS, Nelson C, Waldron PR, et al. Serious bacterial infections acquired during treatment of patients given a diagnosis of chronic Lyme disease – United States. MMWR Morb Mortal Wkly Rep 2017;66:607–9. Available at: https://doi.org/https://doi.org/10.15585/mmwr.mm6623a3. Accessed October 1, 2018.

Diagnosis and Management of Hepatitis B and C

Michelle Pardee, DNP, FNP-BC

KEYWORDS

- Hepatitis B • Hepatitis C • Chronic hepatitis B • Liver disease • Cirrhosis

KEY POINTS

- Hepatitis B and C continue to be public health concerns, causing liver damage, cirrhosis, hepatocellular carcinoma, and death.
- Vaccination is the best way to prevent hepatitis B infection, whereas preventing hepatitis C is accomplished by reducing risk factors.
- Acute hepatitis B and C typically produce minimal symptoms and spontaneously resolve.
- Medication treatments for chronic hepatitis B and hepatitis C can result in remission.

INTRODUCTION

Hepatitis B and C remain common major public health problems worldwide. They can lead to chronic liver disease, cirrhosis, and hepatocellular carcinoma (HCC).[1,2] A global estimate in 2015 indicated 257 million people living with chronic hepatitis B virus (HBV) infection, and 71 million people with chronic hepatitis C virus (HCV) infection.[3] This has prompted member countries of the World Health Organization to set a goal of a 65% reduction in mortality and a 90% reduction in incidence compared with the 2015 baseline,[3] by 2030. In the United States, an estimated 2.2 million people are living with chronic HBV and 3.5 million with chronic HCV.[4] Vaccination programs have significantly reduced the prevalence of hepatitis B, although an estimated actual 20,900 new cases of hepatitis B occurred in the United States in 2016.[4] According to the Centers for Disease Control and Prevention (CDC),[4] the estimated actual new cases of HCV in the United States were 41,200, even with novel treatments for those already infected.

Although hepatitis B and C both cause inflammation of the liver, there are differences in transmission, duration of infection, and treatment options.

HEPATITIS B

HBV causes hepatitis B infection of the liver. Transmission occurs by blood, semen, or other body fluid from an infected individual to an uninfected individual.[4,5] This can

The author has no affiliations or financial relationships to disclose.
The University of Michigan School of Nursing, 426 North Ingalls, #4130, Ann Arbor, MI 48109, USA
E-mail address: milopa@med.umich.edu

https://doi.org/10.1016/j.cnur.2019.02.004
0029-6465/19/© 2019 Elsevier Inc. All rights reserved.

nursing.theclinics.com

occur through sexual contact, sharing needles or syringes, or vertically from an infected mother to baby at birth.[4,5] Hepatitis B can be an acute, short-term illness, although it can become a chronic infection for others.[4,5] Age at acute infection affects the risk of developing chronic hepatitis B (CHB), which can lead to cirrhosis or liver cancer.[1] Infants develop CHB at a far greater rate than those infected as adults.[1,2] Vaccination is the best way to prevent hepatitis B infection, and has dramatically reduced the incidence since universal vaccination of newborns began in the early 1990s.[2,5]

Many people with an acute HBV infection may be asymptomatic, whereas others will have mild symptoms (**Box 1**) and rarely fulminant hepatitis.[6] Risk factors for contracting hepatitis B (**Box 2**) are established, and guide decisions regarding whom to screen for HBV.[1,7,8] The American Association for the Study of Liver Disease (AASLD) recommends in their 2018 practice guidance, to screen for HBV in the following[9]:

- People born in countries with hepatitis B surface antigen (HBsAG) seroprevalence of $\geq 2\%$
- People born in the United States but not vaccinated as an infant, whose parents were born in regions with high HBV endemicity
- Pregnant women
- People needing immunosuppressive therapy
- People in at-risk groups (see **Box 2**)

HEPATITIS B SEROLOGY

Results of serologic assays determine the diagnosis of hepatitis B (**Table 1**).[10] These results also determine acute versus chronic infection, the viral load, or immune status. AASLD hepatitis B guidance recommends using HBsAG and hepatitis B antibody (anti-HBs).[7] A positive HBsAG is the hallmark finding for hepatitis B infection and is detectable 1 to 10 weeks after exposure. In CHB, the HBsAG persists for more than 6 months.[1,7,11] The goal of therapy (if indicated) is for a decline and ultimately negative HBsAG.[11] Anti-HBs indicates immunity, from resolution of an acute infection or vaccination. A negative anti-HBs indicates that the individual is not immune and requires vaccination.[7]

Box 1
Signs and symptoms of hepatitis B

When present, signs and symptoms of acute hepatitis B virus infections can include the following:
- Fever
- Fatigue
- Loss of appetite
- Nausea
- Vomiting
- Abdominal pain
- Dark urine
- Clay-colored bowel movements
- Joint pain
- Jaundice

Data from CDC.gov. What are the signs and symptoms of HBV infection? 2018. Available at: https://www.cdc.gov/hepatitis/hbv/hbvfaq.htm#b7. Accessed October 14, 2018; and CDC. What are the signs and symptoms of acute HCV infection? Available at: https://www.cdc.gov/hepatitis/hcv/hcvfaq.htm#section2. Accessed October 14, 2018.

Box 2
Risk factors for hepatitis B

- People born in Asia, Africa, Middle East, South Pacific Islands, South America, Eastern Europe, Mediterranean
- US-born persons not vaccinated as infants whose parents were born in high-risk regions
- Household and sexual contacts of hepatitis B surface antigen (HBsAG)-positive persons
- Infants born to HBsAG-positive mothers
- Men who have sex with men
- Intravenous drug user
- Multiple sexual partners
- Inmates of correctional facilities
- Renal dialysis
- Health care and public service workers exposed to blood and blood contaminated body fluids
- Unvaccinated persons who travel to countries with endemic hepatitis B

Data from Refs.[1,7,8]

CHRONIC HEPATITIS B

The diagnostic criteria of CHB include the presence of HBsAG for 6 months and includes measuring levels of HBV-DNA, hepatitis B e antigen (HBeAG), and serum alanine transaminase (ALT) to determine infectivity, and liver biopsy to assess liver disease.[7,12] Many with CHB are asymptomatic unless they develop cirrhosis, jaundice,

---

Table 1
Hepatitis B virology and serologic assays

Test		
HBsAG (hepatitis B surface antigen)	Indicates presence of infection	Diagnosis of acute infection Chronic infection if present at least 6 mo
Anti-HBc (HBcAb) (hepatitis B core antibody)	Appears at onset of symptoms in acute infection, persists for life	Indicates previous or ongoing infection in undefined time frame
Anti-HBs (HBsAB) (hepatitis B surface antibody)	Develops as response to vaccination or seroconversion of HBsAG during course of infection or from therapy	Indicates immunity
HBV-DNA	Correlates with levels of HBV virus particles	Stage phase of chronic infection and monitor therapy
HBeAG (hepatitis B e antigen)	Marker of active virus replication	Indicates infectivity
Anti-HBe (HBeAB) (hepatitis B e antibody)	Develops with loss of HBeAG	Remission of disease or inactive Low infectivity

Data from Refs.[1,5,7,9,11]

coagulopathy, ascites, or encephalopathy.[1] The long-term impact of chronic liver inflammation is what leads to cirrhosis and liver cancer.[7] CHB is a dynamic infection and individuals can transition through different phases depending on viral-host mechanisms with variable serology results, viral activity, and infectivity.[1,7]

The initial phase is immune-tolerant CHB and is when HBV is active with minimal disease, although highly infective.[7,12] At this time, HBsAG and HBeAG are positive, with a high level of HBV-DNA and normal or minimally elevated liver enzymes (alanine aminotransferase [ALT] and/or aspartate aminotransferase [AST]).[7,12] The second phase, when the host loses tolerance, is immune-active CHB and is characterized by positive HBsAG, HBeAG, elevated HBV-DNA and ALT and/or AST, causing active liver disease and inflammation that can lead to fibrosis.[7,12] Remission or complete recovery of disease is most common during the immune-active phase and is a negative HBsAG and positive anti-HBs with undetectable HBV-DNA and a normal ALT and/or AST.[7] Inactive CHB can follow after seroconversion of HBeAG to negative and a positive anti-HBe, with an accompanying reduction of viral activity (reduced HBV-DNA) and liver inflammation indicated by a normalization of ALT.[7,12] Some individuals with inactive CHB will move to remission; however, those with negative HBeAG and elevated HBV-DNA CHB can have spontaneous reactivation to immune-active disease.[1,7,12,13]

TREATMENT/MANAGEMENT

Because most individuals with an acute hepatitis B infection do not have symptoms and resolve on their own, there is no indicated treatment.[10,14] However, supportive measures, such as abstaining from ethyl alcohol (ETOH), as well as using universal precautions to prevent infection of exposed contacts should be encouraged.[1,7,15] Medications approved to treat CHB (**Table 2**), include interferon (pegylated) and antiviral agents, such as entecavir, and tenofovir.[7,12,16] For those with CHB, the decision to treat or not, with approved medications, varies by individual and considers serology, HBV genotype, and liver enzymes.[13] The goal of treatment is to suppress replication of HBV, and decrease liver damage and fibrosis and progression to cirrhosis, liver failure, and HCC.[12,15,16]

Table 2 Medication therapies for chronic hepatitis B treatment	
Drug	**Potential Side Effects**
Preferred	
Pegylated interferon	Flulike symptoms, fatigue, cytopenia, anorexia, mood disturbances
Entecavir	Lactic acidosis (decompensated cirrhosis only)
Tenofovir dipivoxil fumarate	Nephropathy, Fanconi syndrome, osteomalacia, lactic acidosis
Tenofovir alafenamide	Lactic acidosis
Nonpreferred	
Lamivudine	Pancreatitis, lactic acidosis (high rates of drug resistance)
Adefovir	Acute renal failure, Fanconi syndrome, lactic acidosis
Telbivudine	Peripheral neuropathy, lactic acidosis

Data from Refs.[7,12,16]

HEPATITIS C

HCV causes hepatitis C infection of the liver. Transmission in at-risk individuals (**Box 3**) occurs in contaminated blood products, use of contaminated needles/syringes, and vertically from an infected mother to infant.[8,9,17] Sexual transmission of HCV can occur, although this is a greater chance in men who have unprotected sex with men, including those who are positive for human immunodeficiency virus.[8,9] Intravenous drug use accounts for approximately 60% of acute hepatitis C infections in the United States.[9] The best way to prevent hepatitis C is the avoidance of risk behaviors, especially injecting drugs.[17]

People with newly acquired HCV infection usually are asymptomatic or have mild symptoms (**Box 4**) that are unlikely to prompt a visit to a health care professional.[18] These signs and symptoms can develop within 6 months of a presumed exposure.[8] Some individuals will have an acute infection that resolves, whereas others will progress to chronic hepatitis C, which can lead to cirrhosis, HCC, a need for liver transplantation, or death.[1] The CDC recommends screening those at-risk individuals (see **Box 4**) and a 1-time screening for all adults born during 1945 to 1965, regardless of risk.[19]

HEPATITIS C SEROLOGY

The diagnosis of hepatitis C is made with a positive HCV-antibody, which indicates acute, chronic, or past infection[20] and can be found 4 to 10 weeks after infection.[21] A positive HCV-RNA, which measures viral replication, is detectable as soon as 1 to 3 weeks after infection and confirms the diagnosis of a current hepatitis C infection.[20] The diagnosis of chronic hepatitis C is when HCV-RNA remains positive for longer than 6 months.[8] Genotype testing is recommended in individuals with a current hepatitis C infection to guide treatment decisions.[8]

CHRONIC HEPATITIS C

Although many individuals with an acute hepatitis C infection will spontaneously clear the infection (negative HCV-RNA), approximately 75% to 85% of people will progress to chronic hepatitis C.[17] Hepatitis C is determined to be chronic when the HCV-RNA remains positive for more than 6 months.[8] At that time, a liver biopsy is performed to determine the level of liver damage and fibrosis and is instrumental in treatment

---

Box 3
Risk factors for hepatitis C

- Blood transfusion or organ transplantation before July 1992
- Intravenous drug use (current or history)
- Needlestick exposure
- Human immunodeficiency virus coinfection
- History of incarceration
- Long-term hemodialysis
- Sexual partner with hepatitis C
- Infants born to hepatitis C–positive mothers

Data from Refs.[1,7,8]

Box 4
Signs and symptoms of hepatitis C

When symptoms do occur, they can include the following:
- Fever
- Fatigue
- Dark urine
- Clay-colored bowel movements
- Abdominal pain
- Loss of appetite
- Nausea
- Vomiting
- Joint pain
- Jaundice

Data from CDC. What are the signs and symptoms of acute HCV infection? Available at: https://www.cdc.gov/hepatitis/hcv/hcvfaq.htm#section2. Accessed October 14, 2018.

Table 3
Medications to treat hepatitis C

Drug Class	Drug Name	Genotype	Adverse Effects
Interferons	Interferon Peginterferon	All Genotypes	Neutropenia, thrombocytopenia, anemia, nausea, rash, cough
Ribavirin	Ribavirin	All Genotypes	Anemia
Direct-acting antivirals			
HCV protease inhibitors	Simeprevir Paritaprevir Telaprevir	Genotype I	Anemia, pruritus, rash, photosensitivity, transient increased bilirubin
HCV NS5A inhibitors	Daclatasvir Elbasvir Ledipasvir	All Genotypes	
NS5B RNA polymerase inhibitors	Sofosbuvir Dasabuvir		Fatigue, headache, nausea
Combinations	Elbasvir/Grazoprevir (ZEPATIER) Ledipasvir/Sofosbuvir (Harvoni) Simeprevir/Sofosbuvir Ombitasvir, paritaprevir, ritonavir + dasabuvir Sofosbuvir + Velpatasvir (EPCLUSA)	Genotype 1 or 4 Genotypes 1, 4 Genotype 1 Genotype 4 All Genotypes 1–6 All Genotypes	

Abbreviation: HCV, hepatitis C virus.
Data from The American Association for the Study of Liver Diseases (AASLD), The Infectious Diseases Society of America (IDSA). HCV guidance: recommendations for testing, managing, and treating hepatitis C. 2018. Available at: www.hcvguidelines.org. Accessed October 30, 2018; and Kohli A, Sherman A, Kottilil S. Treatment of hepatitis C: a systematic review. JAMA 2014;312(6):631–40.

decisions.[8] Individuals with chronic hepatitis C can develop extrahepatic manifestations including skin changes, such as purpura and pruritus; rheumatologic, such as myalgia and arthralgia; and sensory and motor neuropathy.[1] Chronic hepatitis C is progressive and can lead to significant fibrosis, cirrhosis, esophageal varices, and HCC.[1,8,20]

TREATMENT/MANAGEMENT

For individuals with an acute HCV infection, care is symptomatic (see **Box 4** for symptoms), including rest, and cessation of ETOH and injectable drugs (if appropriate).[1,9] Anyone diagnosed with hepatitis C should receive education regarding HCV, transmission, ways to prevent further liver damage, and psychological counseling if desired.[1,9]

Those who do not resolve their acute infection need a liver biopsy to determine the severity of liver damage and urgency for treatment.[8] The AASLD and Infectious Diseases Society of America hepatitis C guidance recommends that all individuals with chronic hepatitis C be treated with antiviral medications, unless there is a shortened life expectancy due to nonhepatic liver diseases.[9] Successful treatment is indicated by a sustained virological response (SVR), which is the absence of HCV-RNA 12 or more weeks after completion of treatment.[1,8,9] Treatment for chronic hepatitis C is complex and based on genotype, degree of fibrosis or cirrhosis, prior treatment, medication side effects, and comorbidities.[1,8,9] Available treatment medications (**Table 3**) include pegylated interferon, ribavirin, and direct-acting antivirals, including combination therapies.[8,9,22] More than 90% of those infected with hepatitis C can be cured and achieve an SVR with appropriate treatment.[23]

SUMMARY

Hepatitis B and C continue to be significant health issues worldwide. The CDC estimates that in 2016, approximately 1700 deaths were attributed to hepatitis B and 18,000 deaths attributed to hepatitis C infection in the United States.[4] Mandatory HBV vaccination has dramatically reduced the prevalence of hepatitis B.[4] For those individuals who develop chronic hepatitis B, medications are used to reduce viral replication and liver damage to progress to remission and complete recovery.[12,15,16]

In the United States, the greatest risk of contracting HCV is in those who use injectable drugs,[9] and the best way to avoid infection is to reduce risk behaviors related to transmission.[17] New medications to treat chronic hepatitis C have produced a cure for more than 90% of infected individuals.[23] Overall, assessing, screening, and treating hepatitis B and C will reduce liver damage, morbidity, and mortality.

REFERENCES

1. Duddempudi AT, Bernstein DE. Hepatitis B and C. Clin Geriatr Med 2014;30: 149–67.
2. Kim BH, Kim WR. Epidemiology of hepatitis B virus infection in the United States. Clin Liver Dis 2018;12(1):1–4.
3. World Health Organization. Global hepatitis report 2017 2017. Geneva. Licence: CC BY-NC-SA 3.0 IGO. Available at: http://www.who.int/hepatitis/publications/global-hepatitis-report2017/en/. Accessed October 23, 2018.
4. CDC.gov. Statistics and surveillance 2018. Available at: https://www.cdc.gov/hepatitis/statistics/index.htm. Accessed October 14, 2018.

5. CDC.gov. Hepatitis B 2018. Available at: https://www.cdc.gov/hepatitis/hbv/index.htm. Accessed October 14, 2018.

6. CDC.gov. What are the signs and symptoms of HBV infection?. 2018. Available at: https://www.cdc.gov/hepatitis/hbv/hbvfaq.htm#b7. Accessed October 14, 2018.

7. Terrault NA, Lok ASF, McMahon BJ, et al. Update on prevention, diagnosis, and treatment of chronic hepatitis B: AASLD 2018 hepatitis B guidance. Hepatology 2018;67(4):1560–99.

8. Wilkins T, Akhtar M, Gititu E, et al. Diagnosis and management of Hepatitis C. Am Fam Physician 2015;91(12):835–42.

9. The American Association for the Study of Liver Diseases (AASLD) and the Infectious Diseases Society of America (IDSA). HCV guidance: recommendations for testing, managing, and treating hepatitis C 2018. Available at: www.hcvguidelines.org. Accessed October 30, 2018.

10. CDC.gov. Hepatitis B serology 2018. Available at: https://www.cdc.gov/hepatitis/hbv/hbvfaq.htm#overview. Accessed October 14, 2018.

11. Jackson K, Locarnini S, Gish R. Diagnostics of hepatitis B virus: standard of care and investigational. Clin Liver Dis 2018;12(1):5–11.

12. Tang C-M, Yau TO, Yu J. Management of chronic hepatitis B infection: current treatment guidelines, challenges, and new developments. World J Gastroenterol 2014;20(20):6262–78.

13. Cox NR, Patel K, Tillmann HL. A rationalized approach to the treatment of patients infected with hepatitis B. Mol Diagn Ther 2014;18:203–12.

14. CDC.gov. How is HBV infection treated?. 2018. Available at: https://www.cdc.gov/hepatitis/hbv/hbvfaq.htm#treatment. Accessed October 14, 2018.

15. Trepo A, Chan HLY, Lok A. Hepatitis B virus infection. Lancet 2014;384:2053–63.

16. Ahn JC, Ahn J. Hepatitis B: standard and novel treatment options. Clin Liver Dis 2018;12(1):19–23.

17. CDC.gov. Hepatitis C 2018. Available at: https://www.cdc.gov/hepatitis/hcv/index.htm. Accessed October 14, 2018.

18. CDC.gov. What are the signs and symptoms of acute HCV infection?. 2018. Available at: https://www.cdc.gov/hepatitis/hcv/hcvfaq.htm#section2. Accessed October 14, 2018.

19. CDC.gov. Persons for whom HCV testing is recommended 2015. Available at: https://www.cdc.gov/hepatitis/hcv/guidelinesc.htm. Accessed November 1, 2018.

20. Ansaldi F, Orsi A, Sticchi L, et al. Hepatitis C virus in the new era: perspectives in epidemiology, prevention, diagnostics and predictors of response to therapy. World J Gastroenterol 2014;20(29):9633–52.

21. CDC.gov. Testing and diagnosis; how soon after exposure to HCV can anti-HCV be detected?. 2018. Available at: https://www.cdc.gov/hepatitis/hcv/hcvfaq.htm#section1. Accessed October 14, 2018.

22. Kohli A, Sherman A, Kottilil S. Treatment of hepatitis C: a systematic review. JAMA 2014;312(6):631–40.

23. CDC.gov. What is the treatment for chronic hepatitis C?. 2018. Available at: https://www.cdc.gov/hepatitis/hcv/hcvfaq.htm#section4. Accessed November 3, 2018.

Zika Virus and Pregnancy Concerns

Karen DeCocker, DNP, APRN, CNM

KEYWORDS

- Congenital Zika syndrome • Zika virus • Microcephaly • Prenatal infection
- Birth defect

KEY POINTS

- Zika virus (ZIKV) is a complex and concerning public health problem because the spectrum of potential birth defects continues to broaden. Prenatal identification and diagnosis of fetal injury associated with ZIKV infection remains limited.
- ZIKV primarily spreads through infected mosquitoes. Transmission is also possible through unprotected sex with someone infected by ZIKV. Transmission is possible, even when a person does not show symptoms of ZIKV.
- All families planning a pregnancy and pregnant women in the United States and territories should be educated on the risks and screened for possible ZIKV exposure and symptoms at each prenatal visit.
- Surveillance for 2 years after delivery of all infants exposed in utero is required to screen, detect injuries, and gain an understanding of all potential consequence of exposure.

INTRODUCTION

Infections have unique considerations and potential dire consequences in pregnancy. In the United States, the District of Columbia, US Territories, and the associated states, a reported total of 6846 women with known possible Zika virus (ZIKV) exposure completed their pregnancies from December 1, 2015 to March 31, 2018. Of these women, 283 infants have likely ZIKV-related birth defects and, in addition, there were 17 fetal losses caused by ZIKV-related birth defects[1,2] (**Fig. 1**).

Some infections affect pregnant women differently than in the general population and can cause fetal injury and pregnancy complications. Immune status changes during pregnancy, with proinflammatory as well as antiinflammatory environments at varying gestational stages, makes pregnant women potentially more susceptible to various infections.[3] Some infections require additional screening, surveillance, and possible alternative treatments that are safe in pregnancy. ZIKV is of special concern

Disclosures: The author has no commercial or financial conflicts of interest and does not have any funding sources.
Department of Women, Children, and Family Nursing, College of Nursing, Rush University, 600 South Paulina Street #1080, Chicago, IL 60612, USA
E-mail address: karen_decocker@rush.edu

because much of the consequence of exposure or infection in pregnancy is not yet fully understood. Infection by ZIKV during pregnancy can cause developmental damage to the fetus, and the altered immune response during pregnancy could possibly be a contributing factor to the change in disease process during ZIKV infection.[3]

Although more is being learned, the extent of varied and less obvious forms of possible fetal damage caused by ZIKV infection during pregnancy is not well understood. New studies have shown damage to the eyes, hearing, and growth, as well as developmental delays. Therefore, education, screening, testing, and consistent reevaluation must be implemented by all care providers and health educators on the risks of ZIKV. Surveillance of all infants from birth to 2 years with suspected or known ZIKV exposure in utero is necessary to catch issues that may be aided with early intervention as well as to learn more about the disease process and the effects long term.[3,4]

Outcomes for US States and the District of Columbia

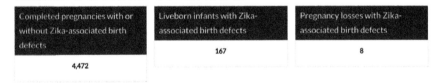

Completed pregnancies with or without Zika-associated birth defects	Liveborn infants with Zika-associated birth defects	Pregnancy losses with Zika-associated birth defects
2,374	116	9

As of **July 17, 2018**, a total of **11** additional completed pregnancies with or without Zika-associated birth defects in the US States and the District of Columbia have been included since the last reporting date, June 19, 2018.

Outcomes for US Territories and Freely Associated States

Completed pregnancies with or without Zika-associated birth defects	Liveborn infants with Zika-associated birth defects	Pregnancy losses with Zika-associated birth defects
4,472	167	8

As of **July 17, 2018**, a total of **54** additional completed pregnancies with or without Zika-associated birth defects in the US territories and freely associated states have been included since the last reporting date, June 19, 2018.

Fig. 1. Numbers of completed pregnancies, live-born infants with birth defects, and pregnancy losses with birth defects that have been associated with possible ZIKV infection. These outcomes include women who completed their pregnancies from December 1, 2015 to March 31, 2018. (*Adapted from* Centers for Disease Control and Prevention. Outcomes of pregnancies with laboratory evidence of possible Zika virus infection, 2015-2018. 2018. Available at: https://www.cdc.gov/pregnancy/zika/data/pregnancy-outcomes.html. Accessed March 19, 2018.)

CONTENT
What is Zika Virus?

ZIKV is a member of the Flaviviridae family. It is spread primarily by daytime-active *Aedes* mosquitoes. In 2012, researchers identified 2 distinct lineages of the virus: African and Asian strains.[5] ZIKV is related to the dengue, yellow fever, and West Nile viruses. ZIKV has been known to occur within a narrow equatorial belt from Africa to Asia since the 1950s. In 2007, the Yap State, the Federated States of Micronesia, reported the first outbreak of ZIKV outside of Africa and Asia. Subsequent infections of ZIKV in other Pacific islands were not reported until 2013, when this virus reappeared in French Polynesia and then disseminated throughout the Pacific.[6] In 2007 through 2016, the virus spread eastward, across the Pacific Ocean to the Americas, leading to the well-known 2015 to 2016 ZIKV epidemic.[5,6]

The infection, known as Zika fever or ZIKV disease, in most cases, causes no or only a few mild symptoms, similar to a very mild form of dengue fever.[7] Among the minority of people infected, and with symptoms, clinical manifestations of ZIKV infection may include fever, headache, arthralgia, myalgia, and maculopapular rash; however, only 1 of every 4 to 5 people who are infected have any symptoms. There is no specific treatment, only mild over-the-counter pain treatment and rest as needed for symptoms. As of 2018, there are no preventive medications or vaccinations against ZIKV. Infection in adults includes a steep increase in Guillain-Barré syndrome, a neurologic disorder that can lead to paralysis and death.[7]

Because ZIKV can spread from a pregnant woman to her baby, infection can result in microcephaly, severe brain malformations, and vision, hearing and other potential birth defects. The ZIKV epidemic is now in decline, but pregnancies in most parts of the Americas and Caribbean still remain at risk because of the ongoing transmission and the potential for new outbreaks.[1,4] During January 2016, the United States Centers for Disease Control and Prevention (CDC) issued travel guidance for affected countries, including the use of enhanced mosquito precautions, safe sex practices, and guidelines for pregnant women, including postponing nonessential travel.[8]

Why the Concern During Pregnancy?

As with known teratogenic viruses, such as rubella, ZIKV infection of the embryo is more likely to result in severe developmental damage with infection in the first few months of pregnancy; that is, during the rapid, early development of the brain.[3] During the 2015 to 2016 outbreak, it became obvious that ZIKV causes developmental damage, known as congenital Zika syndrome, when it became evident in a significant proportion of newborns from mothers infected during pregnancy. Congenital Zika syndrome refers to a constellation of neurologic disorders associated with ZIKV infection, not exclusive to microcephaly.[3]

The most recent reports indicate that the spectrum of fetal brain injury and spectrum of anomalies associated with ZIKV exposure are broader and more complex than microcephaly alone. It is now known that injuries also include subtler fetal brain malformations as well as ocular injuries.[4] Infection with ZIKV is also the cause of other complications of pregnancy, including preterm birth and miscarriage.[9] Because the brain is not fully developed even at birth, subtler neurologic damage may only become evident later in delayed developmental milestones.[3,4]

It is now understood that eye abnormalities may be the first, or even the only, findings in congenital Zika syndrome even in cases in which there is no microcephaly or other apparent neurologic findings.[4,10] Sensorineural hearing loss has also been noted in 5.8% of infants with microcephaly.[4] Any infant with potential maternal ZIKV exposure during pregnancy should have full eye and hearing examinations irrespective of the presence or absence of central nervous system abnormalities.[4,10]

Active viral infections have been confirmed in the placenta and brains of the preterm fetuses from mothers infected with ZIKV.[3,4] It has become clear that maternal ZIKV infection during pregnancy also causes placental infection.[3,4] ZIKV in the maternal blood must be transmitted across the placenta, and in particular the syncytiotrophoblast.[3] In general, these cells are extremely resistant to infection, at least at the time of pregnancy in humans. Early data show that the cells from human, term placentas, which normally are able to resist infection, expressed the genes associated with antiviral defense but do not express the genes that encode attachment factors linked to ZIKV entrance.[3]

In addition, studies have shown that fetuses with significant damage have viral RNA or protein in the brain. Local placental changes may contribute to fetal disease pathogenesis. However, it seems that the virus must reach the fetal brain for the ensuing central nervous system damage to occur.[3]

The efficiency with which ZIKV evades the early immune response to enable infection of the mother, placenta, and fetus is likely critical for understanding why the infection may be either fulminant or limited.[4] Because of ZIKV complexity, the ability to prenatally diagnose fetal injury associated with ZIKV infection remains limited.[3] ZIKV is so proficient at infecting the placenta and the fetal brain that it may help researchers studying ZIKV and the viruses that are very similar to better predict and how to prevent damage with similar epidemics.[4] Encouraging new studies indicate that fetal growth restriction was detected in most fetuses with congenital ZIKV exposure. It seems that ZIKV imparts disproportionate effects and an unusual femur-sparing pattern of growth restriction, which could potentially provide a new approach to identifying viral injury to the fetus earlier in the pregnancy.[4,11] Fetal body ratios may represent a more sensitive form of screening with ultrasonography biomarkers used to detect viral injury in nonmicrocephalic fetuses, which could potentially identify the long-term risk for complications of congenital ZIKV during pregnancy.[11]

What is Known Now

ZIKV is a nationally notifiable disease. The CDC collects data from all states and territories via health departments by using standard case definitions. In 2017, within the United States, there were 452 symptomatic ZIKV cases reported and, of those, 437 were from reported travelers returning home from known affected areas. Seven were from suspected mosquito bites and the final 8 likely from sexual contact. In the US territories where ZIKV is more often endemic, 666 cases were reported, with only 1 from outside travel returning home, 665 from presumed mosquito bites, and none reported by other means, such as sexual contact (**Box 1**).

Box 1
Final data reported to ArboNET

ZIKV disease is a nationally notifiable condition. Cases are reported to CDC by state, territorial, and local health departments using standard case definitions. Shown here are the final 2017 data reported to ArboNET for ZIKV disease.

US states
- 452 symptomatic ZIKV disease cases reported
  - 437 cases in travelers returning from affected areas
  - 7 cases acquired through presumed local mosquito-borne transmission in Florida (N = 2) and Texas (N = 5)
  - 8 cases acquired through other routes, including sexual transmission (N = 7) and laboratory transmission (N = I)

US territories
- 666 ZIKV disease cases reported
  - 1 case in a traveler returning from an affected area
  - 665 cases acquired through presumed local mosquito-borne transmission
  - 0 cases acquired through other routes

From Centers for Disease Control and Prevention. 2017 case counts in the US. 2018. Available at: https://www.cdc.gov/zika/reporting/2017-case-counts.html. Accessed March 19, 2018.

Much has been learned since the United States outbreak but clinicians still do not know many of the critical pieces in what damage ZIKV has caused and how. In the absence of an available vaccine, developing other prevention strategies is key. It is estimated that it could take months or even years to develop a ZIKV vaccine. For now, prevention of ZIKV infection encompasses environmental tactics, personal measures, and vigilant health care and governmental surveillance and research.

What Can Be Done: Education for All on the Risks of Zika Virus

Travelers

People should be advised to avoid travel to areas with known ZIKV or, if living in or must travel to one of these areas, they should be provided with education on steps to prevent mosquito bites and safe sex practices. As for most other viruses spread by mosquitoes, there are no vaccines or medicines available for ZIKV.

- It is crucial to use insect repellent. When used as directed, Environmental Protection Agency (EPA)–registered insect repellents have been proved to be safe and effective, even for pregnant and breastfeeding women.
- Cover up: wear long-sleeved shirts and long pants.
- Keep mosquitoes outside. Use air conditioning, or window and door screens, and use mosquito nets if necessary.

Even when travelers do not feel sick, they should prevent mosquito bites for 3 weeks after their trip so they do not unknowingly spread ZIKV to uninfected mosquitoes. Further, anyone who has been traveling and had symptoms including fever, headache, muscle and joint pain, and rash must see a health care provider immediately and be sure to share their travel history (https://www.cdc.gov/features/stopmosquitoes/index.html).[12]

Preconception education

Pregnancy planning remains a family decision. However, it is known that a high percentage of pregnancies are unplanned. Therefore, it is strongly recommended that all heterosexual couples living in, or traveling to, areas of active ZIKV transmission be advised about the possible risks of infection overall and particularly during pregnancy. The risks of sexual transmission of the ZIKV must be discussed. If the postponement of pregnancy is elected, consistent use of condoms, along with additional means of birth control, is recommended for women and their male sexual partners who live in or travel to areas with active ZIKV transmission.[13,14]

The first documented transmission through sexual contact was in 2008, when a scientist conducting fieldwork in Senegal became infected with ZIKV just before returning to the United States. On his return home to Colorado, he unknowingly infected his wife through unprotected vaginal intercourse before he became symptomatic. This case was the first known sexual transmission of the disease, which is usually transmitted by insects.[13] Women trying to conceive should restrict all nonessential travel to areas of known ZIKV risk. Partners should be counseled to do the same, because of the risk of sexual transmission.[14]

- ZIKV can be passed through sex from a person with ZIKV to his or her partners. Sex includes vaginal, anal, and oral sex and the sharing of sex toys. ZIKV can be passed through sex even in a committed relationship.
- The time frames in which men and women can pass ZIKV through sex are different, because ZIKV virus can stay in semen longer than in other body fluids.
- Infected people can pass ZIKV through sex even when they do not have symptoms. Many people infected with ZIKV virus do not have symptoms or only have mild symptoms, and they may not know they have been infected.

- ZIKV can also be passed from a person before the symptoms start, while they have symptoms, and after the symptoms end.[14]

Pregnant women

The CDC recommends screening throughout pregnancy and encourages special precautions for pregnant women to protect themselves from ZIKV infection by avoiding travel to areas with known ZIKV. If living in, or needing to travel to, one of those areas, education on steps to prevent mosquito bites and practice safe sex should be provided.[15] Sexual partners of pregnant women living in or returning from areas where local transmission of ZIKV occurs should practice safer sex or abstain from sexual activity throughout pregnancy[9] (**Table 1**).

Women should not travel to an area with risk of Zika Pregnant women should not travel to areas with risk of ZIKV (ie, with documented or likely ZIKV transmission). In 2018, no local mosquito-borne ZIKV transmission has been reported in the continental United States.

What to do if living in or traveling to an area with risk of Zika If a pregnant patient must travel to one of these areas, discussion between patient and health care providers must be frequent, and strictly following steps to prevent mosquito bites and practice safe sex is mandatory.

During travel or while living in an area with risk of Zika People should take steps to prevent mosquito bites.

People should take steps to prevent getting Zika through sex by using condoms from start to finish every time they have sex (oral, vaginal, or anal) or by not having sex during a pregnancy.[8]

During pregnancy is it imperative that women share any information on travel, partner travel, and possible exposures, via unprotected intercourse or otherwise, with their care providers immediately. Maternal education on the proper screening methods for infection and exposures should be a routine part of all prenatal care visits (see **Table 1**). If it is discovered during laboratory screening that there has been an exposure during the pregnancy, proper follow-up testing and reporting are essential. Information on the potential risks to the fetus with confirmed exposures and/or infection is imperative at the time of discovery so all families can make informed decisions on how

Table 1 **Zika screening for pregnant women**	
If You...	**When to be Tested**
Traveled to an area with risk of Zika or had sex with a partner who lived in or traveled to one of these areas Live in or frequently travel (daily or weekly) to an area with risk of Zika	• You should be tested if you have symptoms of Zika or if ultrasonography shows that your fetus has abnormalities that might be related to Zika infection • Routine testing is not recommended for pregnant women exposed to these areas who do not have symptoms. However, your doctor may offer testing based on your individual situation • If you have symptoms of Zika at any time during your pregnancy, you should be tested for Zika • If you do not have symptoms, you should be offered testing at your first prenatal care visit, followed by 2 additional rounds of testing at regular prenatal care visits during your pregnancy

Data from Centers for Disease Control and Prevention. Pregnant women. 2018. Available at: https://www.cdc.gov/pregnancy/zika/protect-yourself.html. Accessed March 19, 2018.

they may choose to proceed with the pregnancy and care. Rigorous surveillance of known infected pregnancies is mandatory to ensure proper care and resources are available to the family and potentially affected newborn.

New parents

Proper referral and enrollment in the US Zika Pregnancy and Infant Registry are mandatory and this is the first step in providing appropriate follow-up and support services for families. Assisting in the planning for the continuation of services for affected infants is a responsibility of the entire health care team. Ongoing surveillance and screening of infants and children born with known ZIKV exposure are informing current practices and research areas to better understand the virus as well as the effects of infection during pregnancy. (https://www.cdc.gov/pregnancy/zika/research/registry.html,[16] https://www.cdc.gov/pregnancy/zika/family/documents/WhattoKnow-Congenital-Zika-Syndrome.pdf.[17]).

ZIKV has been found in breast milk, and there have been several reports of ZIKV transmission and infection in babies that were likely caused by breastfeeding.[18] However, there have been zero reports of long-term health problems in those babies resulting from breastmilk from mothers with ZIKV virus infection. All current evidence suggests that the benefits of breastfeeding clearly outweigh the risk of ZIKV virus spreading through breastmilk. The CDC strongly encourages mothers to breastfeed, even in areas with risk of ZIKV. CDC continues to study ZIKV and breastmilk and updates recommendations as new information becomes available.[18,19]

Zika information for parents is available at https://www.cdc.gov/zika/parents/.

What Can Be Done: Provider Education on Proper Screening and Management of Zika Virus

Screening procedures and information for providers

Clinicians should be prepared to discuss and ask about symptoms. Clinical manifestations of ZIKV infection may include fever, headache, arthralgia, myalgia, and maculopapular rash; however, only 1 of every 4 to 5 people who are infected have any symptoms. Thus, clinical symptom reporting alone is an ineffective screening tool for the relative risk assessment of ZIKV infection in most patients. As previously has occurred with other mostly asymptomatic viral infections that pose perinatal transmission risk (such as human immunodeficiency virus or cytomegalovirus), clinicians must develop, continually reevaluate, and implement rapid, sensitive, and specific screening and diagnostic testing for both viral detection and estimation of the timing of exposure[7] (**Box 2**).

For providers assessing risk in pregnant patients This information is direct, with no changes from the CDC Web site (https://www.cdc.gov/zika/hc-providers/testing-for-zika-virus.html) (**Box 3**).

To begin, first ask the patient about travel to or residence in an area with risk of Zika. Ask about potential sexual exposure, including before and during her current pregnancy. Example questions are shown here:

- Have you traveled during pregnancy?
- Have you lived in an area with risk of Zika during your pregnancy?
- Has your partner lived in or travel to an area with risk of Zika during your pregnancy?
- Did you live in an area with risk of Zika before you became pregnant?
- Did you frequently travel (eg, daily or weekly) to one of these areas before you became pregnant?

Box 2
Key information needed for deciding whether to test and how to interpret serology results

- Pregnant women with possible ZIKV exposure should be asked about their risk for exposure both before and during the current pregnancy. Health care providers should ask about the presence of symptoms of ZIKV disease (eg, fever, rash, arthralgia, and conjunctivitis), and place, duration, and type of travel to assess a woman's potential for exposure to ZIKV and other flaviviruses (eg, dengue or West Nile viruses).

- It is important to ascertain whether a woman had exposure to ZIKV before the current pregnancy because ZIKV immunoglobulin M (IgM) antibodies can be detected for months after an infection. A positive ZIKV IgM result could indicate antibodies from infection before the current pregnancy, thus limiting the ability to distinguish between an infection that occurred before the current pregnancy and one that occurred during the current pregnancy.

- It is important to ascertain whether a woman had exposure to flaviviruses other than ZIKV before the current pregnancy because a positive IgM result might have been caused by cross-reactivity from a previous flavivirus exposure.

- Health care providers and counselors should provide appropriate pretest counseling to inform decisions on whether to test; ZIKV test results should be interpreted within the context of known limitations.

- A negative ZIKV IgM test result, if performed during the recommended time frame, in the setting of a negative ZIKV nucleic acid test (NAT) result, provides some reassurance of absence of ZIKV infection during the current pregnancy. However, a negative ZIKV IgM test result should be interpreted within the context of the limitations of the assay.

- When plaque reduction neutralization testing (PRNT) is indicated and performed during the recommended time frame, a negative PRNT result in the setting of a negative NAT result indicates that there is no laboratory evidence of ZIKV infection.

From Oduyebo T, Polen KD, Walke HT, et al. Update: interim guidance for health care providers caring for pregnant women with possible Zika virus exposure - United States (Including U.S. Territories), July 2017. MMWR Morb Mortal Wkly Rep 2017;66(29):781–93.

If the patient previously lived in or frequently traveled to an area with risk of ZIKV, she may have been infected with Zika before pregnancy, and she may have already developed antibodies against ZIKV. If she was infected before pregnancy, Zika antibody test results during pregnancy might not reveal

---

Box 3
Pregnancy and Zika testing

CDC's top priority for Zika is to protect pregnant women because of the risks associated with ZIKV infection during pregnancy.

CDC has interim guidance for health care providers caring for pregnant women with possible ZIKV exposure. This Web tool is intended to help health care providers apply the updated recommendations for ZIKV testing and interpretation of results for pregnant women with possible exposure to ZIKV.

- This Web tool is intended for health care providers and public health officials in the United States and territories.

- CDC continues to evaluate all available evidence and will update recommendations as new information becomes available.

From Center for Disease Control and Prevention. Zika and pregnancy: testing and follow-up on Zika and pregnancy. Available at: https://www.cdc.gov/pregnancy/zika/testing-follow-up/index.html. Accessed March 10, 2019.

whether she was infected in the past or was infected recently during her current pregnancy.

Action needed Ask pregnant women about possible exposure to ZIKV, both before and during the current pregnancy, to help interpret Zika antibody test results and provide appropriate counseling before and after testing. Counseling of families includes a discussion of the limitations of the tests and the potential risks of misinterpretation of test results, including false-positives and false-negatives.

Interpretation of Zika virus testing for providers
The CDC has many resources that are continuously updated on the process for ordering serologic testing. As more information becomes available on the sensitivity and specificity of these laboratory testing methods, the order and process of when and how to collect will continue to be refined (see **Box 2**). In addition, continuing research points to the use of ultrasonography to detect restrictions in fetal growth and monitor growth and femur length as a method of early identification.[11]

SUMMARY

Studies to determine the limitations of prenatal and postnatal testing for detection of ZIKV-associated birth defects and long-term neurocognitive deficits are needed to improve guiding and counseling for women with a possible infectious exposure.[4] Health care personnel must follow CDC recommendations closely and remain up to date on all developments, research findings, and emerging guidelines for testing in women of childbearing age.

How the altered maternal immune response during pregnancy contributes to disease during ZIKV infection is an important area for further investigation. Identifying immune markers associated with the development of (or protection from) microcephaly and other central nervous system defects will be valuable in determining the critical immune processes during infection.[3] As more children are born in areas where ZIKV epidemics have occurred, and diagnostic tests become better able to differentiate ZIKV from other flavivirus infections, especially dengue, a complete clinical picture of the outcomes associated with congenital ZIKV infection will undoubtedly emerge.[3]

All countries in which mosquitoes of the genus *Aedes* are present remain a potential location for future ZIKV outbreaks. These areas includes southern Europe, the Americas, and the Caribbean. Overall, ZIKV outbreaks represent a potentially damaging or even lethal threat to fetuses. There remain significant variations between countries and regions within countries in how this disease trends, and it continues to put large numbers of women at risk with potential outbreaks. Use of governmental and public health resources with the focus on research and prevention is continuously needed. Accelerating the work for vaccine development is a clear priority.[20]

The burden of disease prevention should not be placed exclusively on women of childbearing age. However, the risks and prevention strategies need to be communicated to them in an effective manner (**Box 4**). Family planning, pregnancy screening, and management are critical issues that should be discussed with all at-risk individuals and families. Reproductive and pediatric health care providers and related agencies must work diligently to inform the most vulnerable populations (pregnant women and women of childbearing age and their exposed infants) of the risks ZIKV poses to fetuses/newborns while minimizing parental alarm and anxiety.[20]

Box 4
Helpful links

CDC Zika testing guidelines for providers: https://www.cdc.gov/zika/hc-providers/testing-for-zika-virus.html

Key Zika facts from the World Health Organization: http://www.who.int/en/news-room/fact-sheets/detail/zika-virus

Zika information for parents: https://www.cdc.gov/zika/parents/

Information for parents of babies born with congenital Zika syndrome (PDF): https://www.cdc.gov/pregnancy/zika/family/documents/WhattoKnow-Congenital-Zika-Syndrome.pdf

CDC tracking of Zika in pregnant women and infants: https://www.cdc.gov/pregnancy/zika/research/documents/ZikaRegistry012.pdf

Mosquito prevention information: https://www.cdc.gov/features/stopmosquitoes/index.html

---

REFERENCES

1. Centers for Disease Control and Prevention. 2017 case counts in the US 2018. Available at: https://www.cdc.gov/zika/reporting/2017-case-counts.html. Accessed March 19, 2018.
2. Centers for Disease Control and Prevention. Outcomes of pregnancies with laboratory evidence of possible Zika virus infection, 2015-2018 2018. Available at: https://www.cdc.gov/pregnancy/zika/data/pregnancy-outcomes.html. Accessed March 19, 2018.
3. King NJC, Teixeira MM, Mahalingam S. Zika virus: mechanisms of infection during pregnancy. Trends Microbiol 2017;25(9):701–2.
4. Walker CL, Little ME, Roby JA, et al. Zika virus and the non-microcephalic fetus: why we should still worry. Am J Obstet Gynecol 2019;220(1):45–56.
5. World Health Organization. The history of Zika virus 2017. Available at: http://www.who.int/emergencies/zika-virus/history/en/. Accessed March 19, 2018.
6. Cao-Lormeau V-M, Musso D. Emerging arboviruses in the Pacific. Lancet 2014; 384(9954):1571–2.
7. Eppes C, Rac M, Dunn J, et al. Testing for Zika virus infection in pregnancy: key concepts to deal with an emerging epidemic. Am J Obstet Gynecol 2017;216(3): 209–25.
8. Centers for Disease Control and Prevention. Pregnant women 2018. Available at: https://www.cdc.gov/pregnancy/zika/protect-yourself.html. Accessed March 19, 2018.
9. World Health Organization. Zika virus 2018. Available at: http://www.who.int/en/news-room/fact-sheets/detail/zika-virus. Accessed March 19, 2018.
10. Zin AA, Tsui I, Rossetto J, et al. Screening criteria for ophthalmic manifestations of congenital Zika virus infection. JAMA Pediatr 2017;171(9):847–54.
11. Walker CL, Merriam AA, Ohuma EO, et al. Femur-sparing pattern of abnormal fetal growth in pregnant women from New York City after maternal Zika virus infection. Am J Obstet Gynecol 2018;219(2):187.e1-20.
12. Centers for Disease Control and Prevention. Prevent mosquito bites 2018. Available at: https://www.cdc.gov/features/stopmosquitoes/index.html. Accessed March 19, 2018.
13. Foy BD, Kobylinski KC, Chilson Foy JL, et al. Probable non-vector-borne transmission of Zika virus, Colorado, USA. Emerg Infect Dis 2011;17(5):880–2.

14. Petersen EE, Meaney-Delman D, Neblett-Fanfair R, et al. Update: interim guidance for preconception counseling and prevention of sexual transmission of Zika Virus for persons with possible Zika virus exposure - United States, September 2016. MMWR Morb Mortal Wkly Rep 2016;65(39):1077–81.
15. Centers for Disease Control and Prevention. Guidance for US laboratories testing for Zika virus infection 2017. Available at: https://www.cdc.gov/zika/laboratories/lab-guidance.html. Accessed March 19, 2018.
16. Centers for Disease Control and Prevention. US Zika pregnancy and infant registry. 2018. Available at: https://www.cdc.gov/pregnancy/zika/research/registry.html. Accessed March 19, 2018.
17. Centers for Disease Control and Prevention. What to know if your baby was born with congenital Zika syndrome. 2016. Available at: https://www.cdc.gov/pregnancy/zika/family/documents/WhattoKnow-Congenital-Zika-Syndrome.pdf. Accessed March 19, 2018.
18. Blohm GM, Lednicky JA, Marquez M, et al. Evidence for mother-to-child transmission of Zika virus through breast milk. Clin Infect Dis 2018;66(7):1120–1.
19. Centers for Disease Control and Prevention. Parents. 2018. Available at: https://www.cdc.gov/zika/parents/index.html. Accessed March 19, 2018.
20. World Health Organization. Zika virus and complications: questions and answers 2017. Available at: http://www.who.int/features/qa/zika/en/. Accessed March 19, 2018.

Emerging Infectious Diseases

Donna Behler McArthur, PhD, FNP-BC, FNAP[a,b,]*

KEYWORDS

- Emerging infections • Zoonotic diseases • Vector-borne diseases • *Candida auris*
- *Elizabethkingia anopheles* • Avian influenza • *mcr*-1

KEY POINTS

- Most emerging infectious diseases (EID) are caused by zoonotic pathogens.
- Vector-borne diseases are a major public health problem in the United States.
- Factors contributing to EID include population growth, spread in health care facilities, aging population, global travel, and changing vector habitats related to climate change.

INTRODUCTION

Emerging infectious diseases (EID) are defined as infectious diseases that are newly recognized in a population or have existed but are rapidly increasing in incidence or geographic range. Simply put, they may be new infections resulting from changes or evolution of existing organisms, known infections spreading to new geographic areas or populations, previously unrecognized infections appearing in areas undergoing ecologic transformation, or old infections reemerging because of antimicrobial resistance in known agents or breakdowns in public health measures.[1,2] Emerging infections account for at least 15% of all human pathogens according to the 10th International Conference on EID.[3] A major concern is the synergistic communication between emerging diseases and other infectious and noninfectious conditions. Many emerging diseases are zoonotic or synoptic, an animal receptacle incubates the organism with random transmission into human populations. Likewise, EID may be foodborne, vector-borne, or airborne. Regardless, for an EID to become established, the infectious agent must be introduced into a vulnerable population, and the agent must have the ability to spread from human to human and cause disease.[4]

Disclosure statement: There are no commercial or financial conflicts of interest.
[a] University of Arizona College of Nursing and Department of Neurology, College of Medicine, 1305 North Martin Avenue, Tucson, AZ 85721, USA; [b] Vanderbilt University School of Nursing, 461 21st Avenue South, Nashville, TN 37240, USA
* University of Arizona College of Nursing and Department of Neurology, College of Medicine, 1305 North Martin Avenue, Tucson, AZ 85721.
E-mail address: dbmcarth@email.arizona.edu

In contrast to other human diseases, infectious diseases may be unpredictable with the potential for global outbreaks. Although they are transmissible, there is the potential for immunity against reinfection. Many are preventable through vaccines with the potential for eradication. There is interdependence on nature and human behavior.[5] The challenge of EID relates to their impact on humans: pandemics, epidemics as well as the threats to human health and global stability.[5,6] It is known that the appearance of new infections is inevitable. That said, despite the advances in the development of countermeasures diagnostics, therapeutics, and vaccines, world travel and increased global interdependence have added to problems in diagnosing and containing these diseases. Most can relate to the human immunodeficiency virus (HIV)/AIDS, severe respiratory syndrome, and pandemics, such as the 2009 H1N1 influenza as emerging infections in modern day. The societal and economic impact of these diseases was phenomenal, not to mention the quality of life among infected individuals and their families. Understanding the categories of infectious diseases is important. Specific categories include those that are newly emerging, those that have become established and may periodically reemerge, and those that have become stably endemic.[5,6]

ZOONOTIC DISEASES

Zoonotic diseases are those diseases transmitted from animals to humans through direct contact or through food, water, or the environment, contributing to 61% of infectious organisms affecting humans.[7,8] Zoonotic diseases may be categorized by their ability to spread among humans through 5 stages ranging from only spread among animals (stage 1) to fully human pathogens (stage 5). **Fig. 1** illustrates the stages through which pathogens of animals evolve to cause human diseases.[9]

The National Center for Emerging and Zoonotic Infectious Diseases (NCEZID) aims to protect people from domestic and global health threats. Their scope is broad to include foodborne and waterborne illnesses, infections that spread in hospitals, infections that are resistant to antibiotics, deadly diseases like Ebola and anthrax, illnesses that affect immigrants, migrants, refugees, and travelers, diseases caused by contact with animals, and diseases spread by mosquitoes, ticks, and fleas.[10] Clearly, the interface among humans, animals, and the environment invite diseases impacting public health and social/economic well-being of the global population. Consider the driving factors previously noted. The incidence of zoonoses increases when humans live in close contact with animals and when humans encounter animals in new geographic regions. Some examples include Lyme disease (spread by ticks) and salmonella (spread by poultry). One may recall recent outbreaks of Salmonella in shell eggs, chicken products, raw turkey products, and pet guinea pigs.

ONE HEALTH STRATEGY

The One Health concept began as an initiative among multiple disciplines in 2006. One Health is a collaborative local and global effort to achieve the best health for people, animals, and the environment.[11]

The Centers for Disease Control and Prevention (CDC) uses the One Health approach by working with health care providers, veterinarians, ecologists, and others to monitor and control public health threats and to learn how diseases spread among people, animals, and the environment.[12] The opportunity for nurses to embrace the One Health approach in community and patient education is exponential, for example, working as part of an interprofessional team to educate youth residing in rural

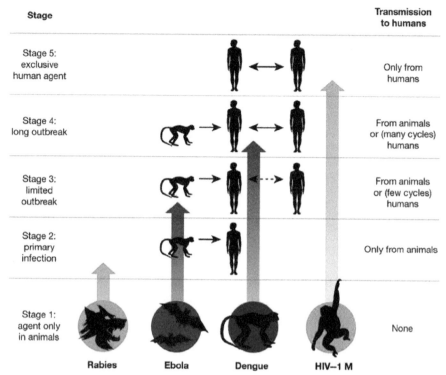

Fig. 1. The 5 stages through which pathogens of animals evolve to cause diseases confined to humans. (*Reprinted from* Wolfe ND, Dunavan CP, Diamond J. Origins of major human infectious diseases. Nature 2007;447:281, Nature/Springer; with permission.)

agricultural areas about preventing the spread of diseases shared between people and animals. There are One Health teams working with 4-H and Future Farmers of America groups. Likewise, the One Health teams educate Americans about diseases they may get from their pets, such as *Salmonella* infections.

VECTOR-BORNE EMERGING INFECTIOUS DISEASES

As alluded to previously, vectors are blood-feeding insects and ticks capable of transmitting pathogens between hosts.[13] These diseases are major causes of mortality and morbidity globally. In the United States, the most common pathogens are transmitted by ticks and mosquitoes, including Lyme disease, Rocky Mountain spotted fever, West Nile, dengue, and Zika virus diseases. These diseases represent a growing public health problem for the United States and globally. Data are tracked by local and state health departments; however, national improvement in surveillance, diagnostics, reporting, and vector control as well as new vaccines has been identified.[13] Mosquito-transmitted EID can spread locally in the United States due to the presence of the specific vector. Likewise, global travel and immigration can bring these infections to the United States with potential transmission.[14] Four mosquito-borne viruses of concern are Zika virus, yellow fever, chikungunya virus, and dengue virus[8,14–17] (**Table 1**). The author refers the reader to the discussion of the Zika virus elsewhere in this journal.

Table 1
Mosquito-borne viral emerging infectious diseases

Name	Epidemiology	Transmission	Clinical Manifestations	Diagnosis	Management	Prevention
Yellow fever	Endemic in sub-Saharan Africa, Central & South America & Caribbean; endemic in 47 different countries. In United States, all cases imported & in unimmunized travelers to risk areas. True incidence unknown due to lack of surveillance	Zoonotic infection spread by mosquitoes in Americas A aegypti. Potential for rapid spread by international travelers. Mosquitoes acquire the virus by feeding on infected primates (human or nonhuman) transmitting virus to other primates. People infected with yellow fever virus are viremic shortly before the onset of fever and up to 5 d after onset. Yellow fever virus has 3 transmission cycles: jungle (sylvatic), intermediate (savannah), and urban. The urban cycle involves transmission of the virus between humans and mosquitoes, primarily. Virus brought to the urban setting by a viremic human who was infected in the jungle or savannah	Incubation 3–6 d. Wide spectrum including asymptomatic. Early flulike symptoms: fever, malaise, myalgia, headache, vomiting. Majority will have bimodal disease. Fever returns within 24 h: hepatitis, jaundice, renal failure. In severe cases, hemorrhage & shock. Among those who develop severe disease, 30%–60% die. Most people with the initial symptoms improve within 1 wk. Residual weakness and fatigue might last several months	Yellow fever infection is diagnosed based on laboratory testing, symptoms, and travel history. Difficult in early phase: confused with malaria and other Flaviviruses	Supportive & symptomatic care. Avoid certain medications, such as aspirin or other nonsteroidal anti-inflammatory drugs, which increase the risk of bleeding. No specific antiviral treatment. IV gamma globulin in early infection. WHO considers confirmed case as seminal event indicating transmission: mass vaccination is required. Issue is not enough vaccine. Vaccine-sparing strategies to immunize enough people for herd immunity & population protection	Control of vector & prevention of mosquito bites. Use Environmental Protection Agency–registered insect repellents, for example, DEET, Picaridin. One vaccine yellow fever–Vax (Sanofi Pasteur, Swiftwater, PA, USA) approved by Food and Drug Administration in United States (www.cdc.gov/vaccines). CDC & WHO recommend those traveling and living in endemic areas receive 1 dose

| Chikungunya virus Ramachandran et al,[16] 2016 & Rathore et al,[14] 2017 | Endemic to Africa & Asia | Arbovirus like Zika, yellow fever, and dengue transmitted by mosquito (A aegypti) (see previous discussion on yellow fever). Recent outbreaks in Europe and Americas (including United States) | Can cause infections in adults & children. Up to 28% asymptomatic. Incubation 3–7 d. Abrupt onset high fever for up to 2 wk, severe polyarthralgia, transient skin rash maculopapular on trunk and extremities. Relapse may occur 2–3 mo after onset. At risk are older adults (>65), persons with comorbidities, neonates exposed intrapartum. Infants & children high risk of atypical or severe disease, for example, vesiculobullous lesions, neurologic complications | Differential diagnosis, dengue fever, malaria, leptospirosis, group A streptococcus, rubella, measles, parvovirus Laboratory tests combined with history. In United States, laboratory test at CDC. Rely on detection of the virus | No specific antiviral treatment Supportive management. Only acetaminophen for joint pain & fever until determined is not dengue fever | Focus on vector control and avoiding further bites to humans to disrupt mode of transmission of infection (see previous discussion on yellow fever) No licensed vaccine for virus, although WHO is evaluating several |

(continued on next page)

Table 1
(continued)

Name	Epidemiology	Transmission	Clinical Manifestations	Diagnosis	Management	Prevention
Dengue virus	Global arboviral Endemic in more than 120 countries, for example, SE Asia & Western Pacific areas, Caribbean, Latin America, some regions of the United States, Africa, Middle East 3.9 billion at risk worldwide. In 2016, large outbreaks worldwide affecting children and adults. Epidemics in the United States in eighteenth and early twentieth centuries. Reemerged in 2016 (Texas & Hawaii) –764 confirmed cases	Transmitted by *Aedes* genus of mosquito (primarily *A aegypti*) Four antigenically distinct virus serotypes, all RNA viruses belonging to Flavivirus (also includes yellow fever, West Nile, Zika, among others)	WHO defines in terms of complexity: without warning signs (fever with nausea/vomiting; rash, myalgias); with warning signs (in addition to above, abdominal pain, clinical fluid accumulation, lethargy); severe dengue (all of the above with severe plasma leakage, severe bleeding)	Confirmatory tests: viral antigen or nucleic acid detection & serology. Difficult to distinguish clinically from Zika & chikungunya virus infections	No specific antiviral agent. Fluid therapy	Tetravalent vaccine approved in some countries, for example, Mexico WHO recommends: Remove all sources of stagnant water to prevent mosquito breeding Prevent mosquito bites: wear appropriate clothing, use of insecticides (see yellow fever) Use of mosquito nets and coils around people sick with dengue fever to prevent mosquitoes biting and transmitting Vector surveillance and control are important

Data from Refs. [8,14–17]

FACTORS CONTRIBUTING TO EMERGENCE OF OUTBREAKS

Three hundred thirty-five EID events were identified between 1940 and 2004. The majority (60.3%) originated from wild animal reservoirs with approximately 1 in 5 transmitted from animal reservoir hosts to humans by disease vectors, for example, ticks and mosquitoes.[18] Fast forward to 2008 and beyond with the discovery of severe fever with thrombocytopenia virus and Middle East respiratory syndrome coronavirus as well as unusual outbreaks of Zika virus, yellow fever, and Ebola. These EID bring to the forefront the significance of demographic change, global travel and trade, and possible climate change as drivers.[2,19]. Biological, social, and environmental drivers, which are interrelated, include the following:

- Microbial adaptation and change (eg, genetic drift and shift in influenza A)
- Susceptibility to infection
- Increased density of human population
- Poverty and social inequality (eg, tuberculosis)
- Stress from farmland expansion on the environment
- Globalization of food market and manufacturing
- Environmental contamination
- Climate change
- Additional opportunities for emerging infections
  - Population growth
  - Spread in health care facilities
  - Aging population
  - International travel
  - Changing and expanding vector habitats (warmer temperatures may allow mosquitoes, and diseases they transmit, to expand to new regions).
  - Drug resistance (contributes to reemergence of bacteria, viruses, and other microorganisms that change over time)
  - Breakdown in public health
  - Intentional biological attacks

A timely example of how these drivers influence emerging diseases is influenza, a causative virus that changes its genetic information. When these changes are marked, the human immune system is challenged and pandemics may occur. The risks of genetic changes and human infection are increased when humans reside near agricultural animals, such as chickens, ducks, and pigs, which are natural hosts of the virus. Avian H5N1 influenza (bird flu) is limited to infection due to direct contact with diseased birds. Although this virus is deadly, it does not have the ability to pass between humans, unlike the H1N1 influenza, which passed into humans from swine. In 2009, this virus reached had a global impact because of human activity, especially air travel.[4]

Another example of an infectious disease attributed to human behaviors is HIV. A leading hypothesis is that humans were first infected with HIV through close contact with chimpanzees, perhaps through bushmeat hunting, in isolated regions of Africa. The spread from rural regions to international regions occurred through air travel. Human behaviors, for example, intravenous drug use, sexual transmission, and transfer of blood products, occurred before the new disease was identified, resulting in rapid spread.[4]

Considering changes in climate, consider the tropical disease of chikungunya (discussed previously). This virus is transmitted by a mosquito originally confined to tropical regions around the Indian Ocean. In 2007, more than 200 residents of a town in Italy suffered from an outbreak of this disease. Subsequently, outbreaks have occurred on all continents.[4]

As health care providers within health care systems, the changing demography of the population merits further discussion. With aging comes the increased risk factors for infection and subsequent hospitalization, adding to the patient's vulnerability. The author discusses the emerging fungal species *Candida auris* causing outbreaks in health care facilities, which is associated with high mortality in patients with underlying comorbidities.[2,20]

NATIONAL INSTITUTE OF ALLERGY AND INFECTIOUS DISEASES EMERGING INFECTIOUS DISEASES CATEGORIES

Not to confuse the reader, but recognizing a resource in the prioritization of emerging pathogen threats to the United States, the author refers to the National Institute of Allergy and Infectious Diseases (NIAID) categorization.[21] **Table 2** highlights the categories with selected examples. NIAID reviews the list in conjunction with federal partners, for example, US Department of Homeland Security and the CDC.

NIAID continues to identify additional emerging and reemerging diseases and pathogens. Within the past 5 years alone, more than 12 diseases and pathogens have been recognized to include *Bordella pertussis*, enterovirus 68, hepatitis C and E, poliovirus, and rubeola.

EMERGING INFECTIONS FROM FUNGUS TO ZOONOTIC FLU VIRUSES

What do *C auris*, *Elizabethkingia anopheles*, the Lone Star tick, and avian influenza H7N2 have in common? They have been identified among the newest emerging infections within the United States. In addition, the plasmid-borne colistin resistance mediated by *mcr-1* (mobilized colistin resistance) may contribute to the dissemination of pan-resistant gram-negative bacteria.[20,22]

Candida auris

An emerging fungal species that is multidrug resistant was identified in 2009 from ear drainage from a Japanese patient. The fungus spread through international travel most notably in New York and New Jersey, causing outbreaks in health care facilities.[20,23,24]

Clinical manifestations of *C auris* include invasive infections with a high mortality from bloodstream infections in patients with serious underlying comorbidities and indwelling devices. Of the 51 persons with the infection in New York from 2013 to 2017,[23] the major concurrent condition (65%) was respiratory insufficiency. The medical intervention noted for most persons was being administered antibiotics within 14 days before the first culture for *C auris*.

The diagnosis can be difficult because of misidentification as another yeast organism. Because of the misidentification, the CDC recommends specific testing methods when select yeast organisms have been reported, for example, *Candida haemulonii*, another emerging drug-resistant strain.[24] Adults should be suspect if they had overnight admissions to health care facilities in affected areas (eg, India, Pakistan, South Africa, Kenya). Clinicians must work with local health departments if infection with this fungus is a possibility.

Management recommendations are outlined by the CDC.[25] Most cases in the United States are resistant to azoles and are susceptible to echinocandin antifungals,

Table 2
National Institute of Allergy and Infectious Diseases emerging infectious diseases/pathogens

Definition	Pathogens
Category A: Organisms/biological agents that pose the highest risk to national security and public health • Can be easily disseminated or transmitted from person to person • Result in high mortalities; potential for major public health impact • Might cause public panic and social disruption • Require special action for public health preparedness	Category A Priority Pathogens • *Bacillus anthracis* (anthrax) • *Clostridium botulinum* toxin (botulism) • *Yersinia pestis* (plague) • *Variola major* (smallpox) and other related pox viruses • *Francisella tularensis* (tularemia) • Viral hemorrhagic fevers: Arenaviruses, Bunyaviruses, Flaviviruses, Filoviruses
Category B: Second highest priority organisms/biological agents • Moderately easy to disseminate • Result in moderate morbidities and low mortalities • Require specific enhancements for diagnostic capacity and enhanced disease surveillance	Category B Select Priority Pathogens • *Burkholderia pseudomallei* (melioidosis) • *Coxiella burnetii* (Q fever) • *Brucella* species (brucellosis) • Ricin toxin (*Clostridium perfringens*) • *Staphylococcus enterotoxin B* • Typhus fever (*Rickettsia prowazekii*) • Foodborne and water-borne pathogens: bacteria (eg, *E coli*, shigella; salmonella, campylobacter); viruses (eg, hepatitis A); protozoa (eg, *Cryptosporidium parvum*, *Giardia lamblia*), fungi • Mosquito-borne viruses (eg, West Nile, yellow fever, chikungunya, Zika)
Category C: Third highest priority. Includes emerging pathogens that could be engineered for mass dissemination in the future because of • Availability • Ease of production and dissemination • Potential for high morbidities and mortalities and major health impact	Category C Select Priority Pathogens • Nipah and Hendra viruses • Additional hantaviruses • Tick-borne hemorrhagic fever viruses (Bunyaviruses, Flaviviruses) • Tick-borne encephalitis complex flaviviruses • Tuberculosis, including drug-resistant tuberculosis • Influenza virus • Other rickettsias • Rabies virus • Severe acute respiratory syndrome associated coronavirus

Data from NIH National Institute of Allergy and Infectious Diseases. NIAID emerging infectious diseases/pathogens. Available at: https://www.niaid.nih.gov/research/emerging-infectious-diseases-pathogens. Accessed July 26, 2018.

which target the fungal cell wall. Cases must be reported immediately to the local public health department.

Prevention begins by being proactive. A response plan for health care staff and environmental services staff should be in place for infection prevention and control of *C auris*. Patients at high risk should be identified within their health care setting, especially if they previously received care in a postacute care setting. Nurses have expertise in assessing patients through comprehensive histories and appropriate physical examinations. Attention should be afforded patients with recent history of health care outside of the United States with known *C auris*.[25]

Elizabethkingia anopheles

This common gram-negative bacillus was discovered in 1959 by Elizabeth King, an American bacteriologist, while working on a bacterium attributed to meningitis in infants. There are 4 species found in soil, river water, and reservoirs worldwide, rarely making people sick. Since 2004, there has been an increased incidence among hospitalized patients, an emerging pathogen.[26,27] The species of concern for this discussion is *E anopheles*, which is known to cause respiratory tract illness in humans.[27] Although the bacteria have been isolated from Anopheles mosquitoes, their role in transmission is unclear.[27] Outbreaks have occurred in Wisconsin,[28,29] Michigan, and Illinois. More than 63 patients have been confirmed with 20 deaths.

Clinical manifestations are more common in immunocompromised patients, those over 65 years, and those with comorbidities. Symptoms include fever, shortness of breath, chills, or cellulitis. The symptoms may mimic an acute viral syndrome; however, if the patient has multiple comorbid conditions (eg, cancer, diabetes mellitus, chronic kidney disease), they should be assessed for *E anopheles*.[27]

Diagnostic criteria include blood cultures. Clinical laboratory tests may be unable to differentiate between *E anopheles* and *Elizabethkingia meningoseptica*. Results should be reported to the state health department as recommended by the CDC, treating presumptively as *E anopheles*.[27]

Management of outbreaks merit immediate antibiotic therapy, especially because septicemia is prevalent. Although *Elizabethkingia* in general is resistant to most antibiotics used to treat gram-negative infections, the patients in multistate outbreaks have been managed with several antibiotics (combination treatment preferred to include fluoroquinolones, minocycline, rifampin, and trimethoprim/Sulfamethoxazole).[20,27,28]

Prevention measures include contact precautions to avoid disease transmission from affected patients to others. The transmission mode is unclear; therefore, conservative precautions should be used for the duration of admission in acute care facilities.[20,27,28]

Lone Star Tick

This aggressive tick, *Amblyomma americanum*, is found in the southeastern, south central, and eastern United States.[20] The distribution and numbers have increased over the past 3 decades. The Lone Star tick does not cause Lyme disease despite the occasional rash in the early stages that may mimic that of Lyme disease.[30]

Disease hosts include deer, for example, wild white-tailed deer, and ground dwelling birds.[20,31] Likewise, the tick will feed on humans and the blood of various domestic and wild animals throughout its lifecycle and can be brought home on pets. A cause of vector-borne diseases, it is associated with the transmission of Ehrlichia, which can cause human ehrlichiosis, heartland virus, tularemia, and southern tick-associated rash illness.[32] In addition, the Lone Star tick may be a vector of the Bourbon virus to humans.[20]

Clinical manifestations usually occur within 7 days after a tick bite with the erythematous rash. The skin lesions are smaller in size than those with Lyme disease (~6–10 cm) and circular in shape with central clearing.[30] Symptoms may include fatigue, fever, headache, joint and muscle pain, but resolve with antibiotic therapy. Heartland virus infections are more common than the Bourbon virus and should be suspected in affected areas when adults present with fever, fatigue, nausea, diarrhea, and anorexia. These individuals do not respond to doxycycline. The Bourbon virus can be fatal in immunocompromised adults and should be included in a differential diagnosis if the patient has thrombocytopenia and leukopenia after a recent tick exposure.

Management is symptomatic with topical corticosteroids for mild local reactions. Doxycycline is the antibiotic of choice.[30]

Prevention includes avoidance measures, for example, for tick habitats: dense woods, brushy areas, use of insect repellent containing DEET (N, N-Diethyl-meta-toluamide) or permethrin, wearing long pants and socks, and performing tick checks with prompt removal.[30] Environmentally, remove leaf debris, which is a source of hydration for the ticks. An interesting recommendation is the importation of fire ants, which serve as a natural means of tick control by eating tick eggs.[31]

Zoonotic Flu Viruses (Not Your Seasonal Flu)

There are 4 types of influenza virus: A, B, C, and D. Type A infects humans as well as many animals. The emergence of new influenza A viruses with the ability to infect people and human-to-human transmission can cause a pandemic.[20,33,34] Persistent influenza threats include the highly pathogenic strains of avian H7N9, H5N1, and H5N6 plus the swine viruses H1N1, H1N2, and H3N2.[20]

Humans can be affected with avian, swine, and other zoonotic influenza viruses. Direct contact with infected animals or contaminated environments is the mode of transmission. Most human cases of influenza A (H5N1) and A (H7N9) are associated with direct or indirect contact with infected live or dead poultry. Seasonal influenza viruses normally circulate in humans in lieu of birds, for example, H1N1, H3N2.[20,35] The avian influenza A (H7N2) is unique in its ability to infect humans in contact with domestic animals.[35] Although the pathogenicity is low and the risk of human transmission is unlikely, the possibility of a widespread problem has to be considered. Influenza in cats spreads the same way as human flu spreads, through direct contact, air droplets, and contaminated surfaces. Germs in cat saliva may be transferred onto the cat's coat during grooming. The virus may manifest through persistent coughing, lip smacking, runny nose, and fever in cats. The overarching concern is animal viruses changing to pose a potential threat to otherwise nonimmune humans. Without existing immunity, outbreaks can occur.[35]

Clinical manifestations following an incubation of 2 to 5 days range from mild upper respiratory tract infection to severe pneumonia, sepsis with shock, acute respiratory syndrome, and death. Individuals at high risk for influenza are the same as those of seasonal flu, for example, children younger than 5, adults 65 and older, pregnant women, people with chronic health conditions, and those who are immunocompromised.[33,34]

Diagnosis is confirmed with laboratory tests using molecular, for example, reverse transcription polymerase chain reaction. Rapid influenza diagnostic tests have lower sensitivity.

Management includes some antiviral drugs (neuraminidase inhibitors), which can reduce duration if prescribed within 48 hours of onset and continued for at least 5 days. Symptomatic treatment is the key.[33–35]

Prevention includes controlling the animal source. Surveillance in animal and human populations is critical (see One Health discussion). Personal protective measures include regular hand washing and proper drying of hands, respiratory hygiene, early self-isolation, and avoid the touching of the eyes, nose, or mouth. All health care providers must use airborne precautions.[33,34]

Travelers to countries with outbreaks of avian influenza should avoid poultry farms, avoid contact with animals in live poultry markets, and practice food safety. Travelers returning from affected regions should report to local health authorities if respiratory symptoms occur.

MCR Genes

Although there is no immediate public threat, mcr-1 brings to the forefront the global challenges in addressing antibiotic resistance and best practices for antibiotic use.[20] The mcr-1 gene causes resistance to colistin, which is considered by the CDC to be a "last resort "antibiotic.[36] Consider the overuse and misuse of antibiotics in humans and animals. The common bacterial infections once treatable have become resistant to other antibiotics or require the last line of antibiotics, which can have serious side effects.[37,38]

The mcr gene is found on small pieces of DNA (plasmids) that carry genetic instructions from 1 bacterium to another, enabling resistance to be shared. One bacterium is carbapenem-resistant Enterobacteriaceae.[36,37] This gene was first identified in November 2015 in China. What is unique about mcr-1 is its potential to spread to other bacteria, some of which may have resistance to major antibiotics and could become resistant to colistin, a last resort option. The CDC and its federal partners continue to track mcr-1 in the United States. In May 2016, Escherichia coli bacteria carrying the gene was found in a urine sample from a patient in Pennsylvania and from intestinal samples of 2 pigs from South Carolina and Illinois. Fortunately, the patient from Pennsylvania was not resistant to all antibiotics. This discovery emphasized the importance of coordinated efforts among the CDC and state and local health departments. The CDC has developed a rapid laboratory test to help clinical laboratories find bacteria with mcr-1.

NURSES' ROLES IN EMERGING INFECTIOUS DISEASES IDENTIFICATION AND PREVENTION

Clinicians recognize that EID are inevitable and unpredictable. Partnering with interprofessional teams, patients, and communities, nurses must become vigilant in acknowledging unusual presentations and seeking appropriate diagnostics. According to the European Society of Clinical Microbiology and Infectious Diseases Emerging Infections Task Force Expert Panel, mathematical modeling has not been able to predict outbreaks. Being knowledgeable about emerging infections increases the ability to include these in differential diagnoses in clinical practice as well as recognizing best practices in care through evidence-based resources. In addition, best practices for self-care should be implemented to include adherence to vaccination recommendations.

Targeted screening for migrants arriving from highly endemic countries can be a front-line defense and can be cost-effective. Preventative vaccinations programs are recommended, concentrating resources on those who need it most. Successful integration of migrants into the local health care system and partnering with public health facilities will ensure better diagnosis and management of diseases.[39]

Nurses' unique skill sets brought to health care settings enhance the ability to assess patients for EID as well as promote health in the community.[28] Each patient history must include a detailed travel history. It is the astute clinician who makes the connection among patient histories and recognizes the first signs of an EID.[19]

Nurses must be current on EID in their geographic areas as well as globally and know where to locate resources in a timely manner, for example, World Health Organization (WHO), CDC, subscribing to medical reference apps.

Selected Resources

http://www.niaid.nih.gov/research/emerging-infectious-diseases-pathogens.
http://wwwnc.cdc.gov/eid.

EID on Twitter (http://twitter.com/CDC_EIDjournal).
Morbidity and Mortality Weekly Report (MMWR) (https://www.cdc.gov/mmwr/).
NCEZID Follow @CDC NCEZID on Twitter (http://twitter.com/CDC_NCEZID).
CDC Vital Signs (https://www.cdPc.gov/vitalsigns/).
http://www.cdc.gov/vaccines/index.html.
http://wwwnc.cdc.gov/travel/destinations/list.

SUMMARY

Emerging and reemerging infectious diseases are difficult to predict, let alone manage. Emerging pathogens include vector-borne diseases, such as the Lone Star virus as well as numerous mosquito-borne diseases. New *Candida* and *Elisabethkinga* infections threaten patients in hospital settings. Recognizing drivers contributing to outbreaks helps shape strategies for health care providers to work together, embracing One Health. Integrating emerging infections into differential diagnoses within practice settings is 1 way to impact patient and community health outcomes.

REFERENCES

1. Centers for Disease Control and Prevention (CDC). National Center for Emerging and Zoonotic Infectious Diseases (NCEZID) NCEZID CD. 2017. Available at: https://www.cdc.gov/ncezid/index.html. Accessed October 2, 2018.
2. Petersen E, Petrosillo N, Koopmans M, ESCMID Emerging Infections Task Force Expert Panel. Emerging infections-an increasingly important topic: review by the Emerging Infections Task Force. Clin Microbiol Infect 2018;24:369–75.
3. CDC International Conference on Emerging Infectious Diseases. Available at: https://www.cdc.gov/iceid/index.html. Accessed August 3, 2018.
4. Baylor College of Medicine. Emerging infectious diseases. Available at: https://www.bcm.edu/departments/molecular-virology-and-microbiology/emerging-infections-and-biodefense/emerging-infectious-diseasesous diseases. Accessed October 3, 2018.
5. Fauci AS, Morens DM. The perpetual challenge of infectious diseases. N Engl J Med 2012;366:454–61.
6. Morens DM, Fauci AS. Emerging infectious diseases: threats to human health and global stability. PLOS Pathog 2013;9(7):e1003467.
7. Ryu S, Kim BI, Lim J-S, et al. One health perspectives on emerging public health threats. J Prev Med Public Health 2017;50:411–4.
8. World Health Organization (WHO). Zoonoses. Available at: http://www.who.int/zoonoses. Accessed October 3, 2018.
9. Wolfe ND, Dunavan CP, Diamond J. Origins of major human infectious diseases. Nature 2007;447:279–83.
10. CDC. National Center for Emerging and Zoonotic Infectious Diseases (NCEZID). 2018. Available at: https://www.cdc.gov/ncezid/index.html. Accessed August 3, 2018.
11. One Health Initiative. Available at: http://www.onehealthinitiative.com. Accessed September 3, 2018.
12. Centers for Disease Control and Prevention. One Health. Available at: https://www.cdc.gov/onehealth/index.html. Accessed September 3, 2018.
13. Rosenberg R, Lindsey NP, Fischer M, et al. Vital signs: trends in reported vector-borne disease cases- United States and territories, 2004-2016. MMWR Morb Mortal Wkly Rep 2018;67(17):496–501.

14. Rathore MH, Runyon J, Haque TU. Emerging infectious diseases. Adv Pediatr 2017;64:27–71.

15. CDC. Yellow fever. 2018. Available at: https://www.cdc.gov/yellowfever/index.html. Accessed October 3, 2018.

16. Ramachandran VG, Das S, Roy P, et al. Chikungunya: a reemerging infection spreading during 2010 dengue fever outbreak in National Capital Region of India. Virusdisease 2016;27(2):183–1286.

17. Centers for Disease Control and Prevention Dengue. Available at: http://www.cdc.gov/dengue/index.html. Accessed October 9, 2018.

18. Jones KE, Patel NG, Levy MA, et al. Global trends in emerging infectious diseases. Nature 2008;451:990–3.

19. Van Doom HR. Emerging infectious diseases. Medicine 2014;42(1):60–3.

20. Bunnell KL. 5 emerging infections to watch out for in 2018. Contagion Live-Infectious Diseases Today. 2018. Available at: https://www.contagionlive.com/publications/contagion/2018. Accessed September 28, 2018.

21. NIH National Institute of Allergy and Infectious Diseases. NIAID emerging infectious diseases/pathogens 2018. Available at: https://www.niaid.nih.gov/research/emerging-infectious-diseases-pathogens. Accessed September 28, 2018.

22. MacNair CR, Stokes JM, Carfrae LA, et al. Overcoming *mcr-1* mediated colistin resistance with colistin in combination with other antibiotics. Nat Commun 2018;9:458. Available at: www.nature.com/naturecommunications. Accessed October 3, 2018.

23. Adams E, Quinn M, Tsay S, et al. *Candida auris* in healthcare facilities, New York, USA, 2013-2017. Emerg Infect Dis 2018;24(10):1816–24.

24. Sears D, Schwartz BS. *Candida auris*: an emerging multidrug-resistant pathogen. Int J Infect Dis 2017;63:95–8.

25. CDC. Candida auris. 2018. Available at: www.cdc.gov/fungal/candida-auris. Accessed September 28, 2018.

26. Yung CF, Maiwald M, Loo LH, et al. *Elizabethkingia anopheles* and association with tap water and handwashing, Singapore. Emerg Infect Dis 2018;24(9):1730–3.

27. Malviya M, Bronze MS. Elizabethkingia infections. 2017. Medscape Website. Available at: https://emedicine.medscape.com/article/2500046-overview. Accessed October 14, 2018.

28. Coyle AL. *Elizabethkingia anopheles:* exploring the outbreak of disease in the Midwest. Nursing 2017;47(3):61–3.

29. Castro CEF, Johnson C, Williams M, et al. *Elizabethkingia anopheles:* clinical experience of an academic health system in Southeastern Wisconsin. Open Forum Infect Dis 2017;4(4):1–4.

30. CDC. STARI or lyme?. 2015. Available at: https://www.cdc.gov/stari/disease/index.html. Accessed October 14, 2018.

31. Reynolds HH, Elston DM. What's eating you? Lone Star Tick (*Amblyomma americanum*). Cutis 2017;99:111–4.

32. CDC. Ehrlichiosis. 2018. Available at: https://www.cdc.gov/ehrlichiosis/index.html. Accessed October 14, 2018.

33. CDC. Seasonal flu vs. pandemic flu. 2018. Available at: https://www.cdc.gov/flu/pandemic-resources/basics/about.html. Accessed September 28, 2018.

34. WHO. Influenza fact sheet. 2018. Available at: http://www.who.int/en/news-room/fact-sheets/detail/influenza-(avian-and-other-zoonotic). Accessed September 28, 2018.

35. CDC. H7N2 questions & answers. 2018. Available at: https://www.cdc.gov/flu/other/flu-in-cats/h7n2-cat-faq.html. Accessed October 14, 2018.
36. CDC. Newly reported gene, *mcr*-1, threatens last-resort antibiotics. 2018. Available at: https://www.cdc.gov/drugresistance/solutions-initiative/stories/gene-reported=mcr.html. Accessed October 2, 2018.
37. CDC. Tracking the mcr gene. 2018. Available at: https://www.cdc.gov/drugresistance/biggest-threats/tracking/mcr.html. Accessed October 2, 2018.
38. Al-Tawfiq JA, Laxminarayan R, Mendelson M. How should we respond to the emergence of plasmid-mediated colistin resistance in humans and animals? Int J Infect Dis 2017;54:77–84.
39. Khyatti M, Trimbitas R-D, Zouheir Y, et al. Infectious diseases in North Africa and North African immigrants to Europe. Eur J Public Health 2014;24(Suppl 1):47–56.

Printed and bound by CPI Group (UK) Ltd, Croydon, CR0 4YY

03/10/2024

01040477-0008